Story Writing
in a Nursing Home:
A Patchwork of Memories

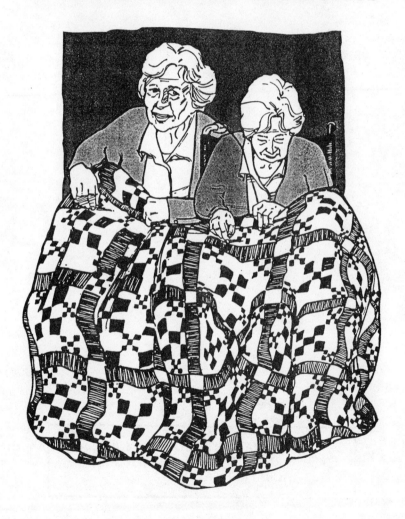

Story Writing
in a Nursing Home:
A Patchwork
of Memories

Martha Tyler John

The Haworth Press, Inc.
New York • London • Sydney

Story Writing in a Nursing Home: A Patchwork of Memories has also been published as *Activities, Adaptation & Aging*, Volume 16, Number 1 1991.

The Haworth Press, Inc. 10 Alice Street, Binghamton, NY 13904-1580
EUROSPAN/Haworth, 3 Henrietta Street, London WC2E 8LU England
ASTAM/Haworth 162-168 Parramatta Road, Stanmore, Sydney, N.S.W. 2048 Australia

Illustrations by Bruce John.

Library of Congress Cataloging-in-Publication Data

John, Martha Tyler.
    Story writing in a nursing home: a patchwork of memories/ Martha Tyler John.
      p. cm.
    "Has also been published as Activities, adaptation & aging, volume, 16, number 1, 1991" — T.p. verso.
    Includes bibliographical references.
    ISBN 1-56024-098-9 (acid-free paper)
    1. Autobiography — Therapeutic use. 2. Aged — Rehabilitation.
RC953.5.J64 1991
615.8'51 — dc20
                                      91-25476
                                       CIP
                                       r91

Story Writing in a Nursing Home: A Patchwork of Memories

CONTENTS

ABOUT THE AUTHOR

Martha Tyler John, EdD, is currently Dean of the School of Education and Human Services at Marymount University. She has been an educator for a number of years and has worked with the frail elderly since 1976 when she began providing mental stimulation for people in the Extended Care facility in Prince George's County, Maryland. Since then she has brought lessons and student volunteers to Indian Hills and Good Samaritan Nursing Centers in Olathe, Kansas, and to Powhatan Nursing Center in Falls Church, Virginia. Dr. John wrote the books *Teaching and Loving the Elderly* and *Geragogy: A Theory for Teaching the Elderly*.

ACKNOWLEDGEMENTS

Martha Tyler John is the author of *Storywriting in a Nursing Home* but wishes to recognize the contributions of other people who have made the book so enjoyable to read. The elderly folks at Powhatan Nursing Center in Falls Church, Virginia and those at Countryside Manor in Loudoun, Virginia wrote and/or told the the stories that are provided in Chapters 3, 4, and 5. The graduate students at Marymount University helped by listening to and recording stories as the older individuals told them. It was necessary for the students to type up the stories and to take the stories back to the writers/ tellers two or three times. The stories needed to be as accurate as possible. Appreciation for the efforts is hereby extended.

Introduction

Powhatan Nursing Home and Countryside Manor have been the center of much activity every Tuesday morning. At about 10:30 a.m. some 30 to 50 patients, family members and staff gather for a learning session. Sometimes, folks have come in a van from Madison Day Center, and they are ready to join in the lessons. The average age of the participants is 86 years and the sense of expectation and enthusiasm runs high. There is no doubt that these people are prepared to learn and share ideas. The topics being studied vary from "endangered species" to "colonial times" to "different cultures" to "computers" and even "the metric system." New vocabulary, discussion questions, games, puzzles, plays, media (filmstrips/tapes, films, slides) and songs all serve to enliven the sessions. Roomwork, (so similar to homework that it is hard to tell the difference) including reading and written responses, is given to provide for follow-up and reinforcement of the ideas the mental stimulation session has presented. Roomwork is reviewed and collected the following week and discussed by the group. A brief recap of the instructional ideas shared the week before is given and a new lesson is begun.

There were several reasons for making a Patchwork Storybook:

1. to provide mental stimulation for elderly people in nursing home settings,
2. to challenge them to record some events of interest from their lives,
3. to preserve these stories of earlier days for a wider audience,

4. to encourage other volunteers to organize and collect ideas from our valuable elderly folks,
5. to demonstrate the way in which college or university students can participate in a practical working relationship with frail elderly people.

Hopefully, this book will demonstrate the ways in which elderly people can be productive and can enrich our lives.

Martha Tyler John

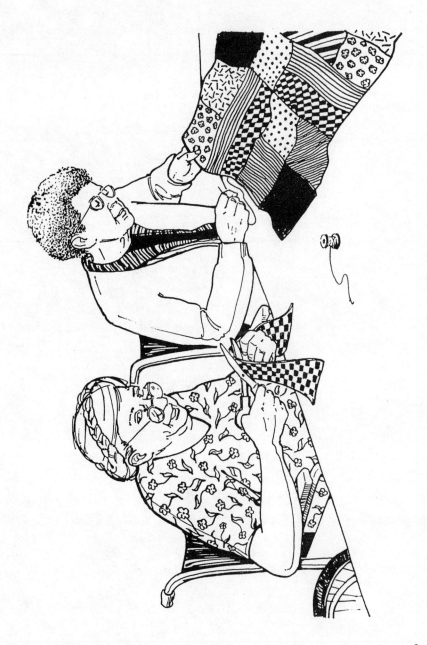

Chapter I

Designing the Quilt

Information about the genesis of this book might be of interest to the reader. *Storywriting in a Nursing Home* was developed as a result of many sessions with wonderful people in nursing centers. During the learning sessions, older adults frequently told stories of events that had happened to them in their youth. They would think of the incidents that related to some particular learning topic and share bits of the idea with the other participants. The teacher would quickly bring the microphone to the person who had a story to tell and would question the teller in some depth so that the listeners could hear the details of an experience that related to the topic under consideration. Without any specific encouragement, some of the participants began to tell stories once in a while. They did not try to dominate the sessions, but would tell about something that related to the topic being considered.

One gentleman who was 95 years old and blind had the most exceptional memory. He was an engineer with a degree from Brown University, and had worked for Franklin D. Roosevelt when F.D.R. was the governor of New York, and before he became president of the United States. Mr. Gumb could tell stories in such a way that the audience was held spell bound. Another man who was in a wheel bed had built a cabin up in the mountains of West Virginia with his son when he had been in good health. His eyes would light up so when he told about this experience that it provided entertainment and a lingering feeling of pleasure for everyone who listened. His children and even his great grandsons came to see him on occasion and took part in the instructioinal sessions. The stories were very interesting and the author decided to try to systematically record the better stories.

THE QUILT FRAME (Background Data)

To help motivate other elderly folks to participate in the learning sessions and encourage them to tell stories, Interest Inventories were taken to determine what they would want to learn about. The Interest Inventory was as follows:

INTEREST INVENTORY

Instructions

Collect the data for each item in a systematic way, however, use an informal, warm approach. Do not crowd the elderly person who is being interviewed. The amount of time needed for a response may be a bit longer than one would anticipate with a heterogeneous population. Remember that the one common descriptor for elderly persons is behavioral slowing.

1. NAME_____

2. FORMER ADDRESS_____

3. BIRTHPLACE_____

4. DATE OF BIRTH_____

5. SCHOOLING_____

6. DID YOU HAVE ANY ESPECIALLY INTERESTING SCHOOL EXPERIENCES?_____
   _____

7. CHILDHOOD GAMES AND ENTERTAINMENT THAT YOU ENJOYED?_____

8. DID YOU HAVE ANY SERIOUS ILLNESSES?_____
   _____

9. WERE YOU IN THE MILITARY SERVICE?_____

10. HAVE YOU TRAVELED? WHERE?_____
    _____

11. DID YOU MARRY? WHEN?_____

12. WHAT WAS YOUR OCCUPATION? YOUR SPOUSE'S OC-
    CUPATION?_____

13. DID YOU HAVE CHILDREN?_____

14. WHEN WERE THEY BORN?_____

15. DO YOU HAVE GRANDCHILDREN/TELL SOMETHING
    ABOUT THEM._____

    _____

    _____

    _____

16. WERE THERE MAJOR PROBLEMS IN YOUR LIFE?

    _____

    _____

17. WHAT SPORTS DID YOU ENJOY OR DO YOU ENJOY
    NOW?_____

    _____

18. DO YOU LISTEN TO RADIO OR TV? WHICH SHOWS?

    _____

    _____

19. WHAT KIND OF STORIES DO YOU READ?_____

    _____

20. DO YOU ENJOY MUSIC? WHAT KIND?_____

    _____

21. DO YOU DO ANY TYPE OF HANDWORK?_____

_____

22. ARE THERE CURRENT ISSUES NATIONALLY THAT CONCERN YOU? NAME THEM._____

_____

Choosing a Design

Based on the results of the inventories a number of topics could be seen to have interest for the elderly participants. They had listed stories about colonial America, information about plants and animals, travelogs, concern for the environment, and an interest in famous Americans both past and present. The interests of the groups were clear and instructional sessions were designed around these topics. Now another step was needed—an emphasis on writing or story telling would be needed to prepare the participants for the production of stories that would be readable and enjoyable for other people.

Therefore, a series of lessons was designed to emphasize different "Types of Stories". Sessions were designed that examined several kinds of stories and showed how to write the story type being discussed. Filmstrips and tapes on each of the following topics were shown and discussed:

> Myths and Legends
> Historic Fiction
> Adventure Stories
> Real Life Stories
> Story Illustrations

Lesson plans and examples of the work that was done on the topics will form the basis for this book. Media, such as filmstrips, movies, video tapes or slides were used to begin each session to set a focus for the topic being considered. Such material would help bring to the mind of the elderly participants information or ideas that may not have been considered for some time.

Learning to Quilt

Providing learning opportunities for the frail elderly in nursing centers is based on an important democratic principle. It is the idea that all people have the right to learn; and, that it is difficult for people to search out new learning experiences for themselves when they are in a physically confining environment such as a nursing home. There are no learning materials prepared specifically for this group of people and the formal school system that is available to younger, more mobile people is not available to them. Special education has not really dealt with the needs of the elderly. Homebound instruction deals with what is thought of as the "normal" age range of students. In effect, very few people seriously consider the learning needs of the very old person.

Because old, older adults do not have formal classes provided, it is possible for those living in nursing homes to become careless about learning. As learning decreases, the brain gets "flabby," and the mental stimulation that accompanies learning is diminished. Reduced mental activity can affect both the physical and mental health of the person. "Challenging your brain to keep it in optimal condition is vital not only to your central nervous system but to your entire body" (Winter & Winter, 1986, p.4). Mental exercise is necessary, and can help older people maintain better physical and mental health. It may also aid them in preserving at least some modicum of independence. Because this is so, learning opportunities need to be designed that allow elderly people to begin gradually to investigate new ideas and to review old experiences.

THE COLOR AND FABRIC
OF PATCHWORK PARTICIPANTS

Aging is a relative thing and what is young in one society may be considered middle aged in another. It was a surprise to the author when carrying out a Fulbright Professorship in Botswana in 1980 to discover that the retirement age for government workers there was 45 years of age. The life expectancy was no where near what it was in the United States at that time. Forty-five was rather old for people who could expect to live only into their fifties. Conversely, there are some cultures such as the Hunza in Pakistan and the Abkhazia in Russia who live to be very, very old by our standards. They live to be well past 100 — many living to be one hundred and twenty to one hundred and thirty years of age. They seem to be active much longer than Americans are, also. In these cultures the social status is high, and family members often live with other members of their families. There is no forced retirement in these cultures, and they carry out tasks in their rural communities with dedication. Many of them are members of a council of elders and make decisions that effect the total community. People in these "long life" communities seem to have a different attitude toward life. They expect to live longer. Their diet is different; they eat less using low calorie diets throughout life. They consume few fats that are of animal origin and maintain a high level of physical activity. Of course, there may be genetic factors involved in this longer life. Their parents lived to be very old and it may be that they do not have the genes that carry the predisposition for fatal or disabling disease. In small communities like these, there is much intermarriage and the genetic pool, whatever it is, would be fairly constant.

However old people in a community live to be, it is important that the wisdom of the elders be utilized. The first step involved in using the wisdom of the elders is to recognize the value of our older population. If this is done, then the need to provide opportunities for them to remain active mentally becomes more obvious. The very old have stored in their vast mental databank of memories, adventures and historic events that would be meaningful to their families and of interest to other people, as well. Much of what is needed is to renew the learning from past years and open up ways for them to organize and share their lives with others.

Older people know what they value, what is worth striving for and how to love. They can provide living symbols of these qualities for the generations that follow them. In addition, they can give us many creative products. The author's mother produced her first book when she was 76; her second when she was 78; her third when she was 83; her fourth at the age of 91; and her fifth book was nearing completion when she died at 94 years and 10 months. It was her fondest wish that this last book, on which she had spent many hours of research, be published. There was still work to be done on the book and, so, the author edited it and her son, Bruce, a professional artist, did the illustrations for Grandma's book which has since been published.

Grandma Moses is an example of another elderly "beginner" who began to produce great paintings late in her life, long after many people would have retired. These paintings provide valuable insights into the quality of life during her lifetime. Other older adults have produced creative paintings, poems and short stories, and these are a source of enjoyment for them and their families and often for the world at large.

Because the creative ability of elderly people is often overlooked, a special session was done with the folks at Powhatan to remind them of their creative, potential, Steps were stressed that indicate what is needed to produce a creative product.

1. Skill is a necessary part of any creative product. The individual may have special skill in using words either in speech or in writing; s/he may be gifted in musical or artistic ability, in working with wood, in inventing any one of a number of objects, or in a variety of other ways.
2. A certain "mind-set" is needed if one is to produce a creative product. The elderly were told that it would take some time to remember the interesting events that they wished to write about; that the individuals recording the stories for them might need them to repeat information more than once; that one or two improvement sessions might be needed if they were to record a really good story. Mind-set, persistence, are essentials in producing any creative product.
3. The products any individuals produce are based on a unique combination of talent and background experience. Some of the elderly folks at Powhatan have had unique experiences that could be of interest to others, but were unable to write the stories due to physical problems. Marymount University students were eager to listen to the stories of the older people, and the combined talents of elders and students make it possible to produce creative stories.
4. Most creative products also have a certain dynamic quality about them. They involve others in the ideas and help the indi-

viduals experience a new idea or a new dimension in their
lives. Our elderly creators were reminded that they needed to
make their stories seem exciting and dynamic so that they involve the reader.

PIECES IN A PATCHWORK

The many colors and fabrics of the pieces in a patchwork quilt
make it bright and interesting. Like the bits that make up the quilt,
older people have had a patchwork of experiences and when these
are put together, they form a colorful background of memory.
These elderly citizens have survivied depressions and wars and can
share with the younger generation the stories of their passage in a
positive, forthright way. Sometimes one can detect a twinkle in the
eye of an older person as s/he tells of a humorous event that occurred in the midst of some very trying time. They have a sense of
acceptance of the passing of time that can bring ease to an individual who is suffering from stress. As a nation, we need the stability
this kind of humor and sharing can give us.

Each story that an older person tells is like a piece of a quilt
block. It may only represent one bit of color or one type of texture;
but put together with other pieces, it can make a beautiful quilt. We
have encouraged the elderly folks at Powhatan Nursing Center to
write or tell stories that will share the flavor of their lives with other
people; that will highlight the texture and color of yesteryear for the
reader of this book of memories.

Many older adults in nursing centers have suffered some trauma
and are somewhat limited in physical capacity, but their memories
are good and their need to communicate is as strong as ever. They
have lived rich, full lives and can remember the most incredible
events; like the lady who remembered being a part of the "living
flag" as a school child when the nation celebrated the 100th birthday of the writing of the Star Spangled Banner. She had to wear a
white blouse, because she was one of the stars in the flag and she
stood on the hill on Fort McHenry's hillside in 1914 with hundreds
of other elementary school children to make this "living flag" in a
service honoring the centennial of The National Anthem. This was

such a vivid memory, and the sense of history memories like this give us provides great continuity for our lives. If people are to gain from the wisdom and the rich memory of the older adult, from their patience and their steady endurance, then some way of sharing these qualities must be designed.

MANAGING THE DIFFICULT STITCHES

There are problems in getting older adults to record memorable events, however. For one thing, many of them do not think the things that happened to them were in any way unique. They will say "Oh, I lived a very ordinary life," or sometimes, "Nothing much ever happened to me." If the stories that are within them are to be recorded, they need to be encouraged to think about the unique, funny, sad or terrifying events that took place in their lives. Once this is done, there can be a rewarding story telling time.

Yet a second problem exists, however. Some frail elderly cannot write well due to stroke or muscular deterioration. If their stories were to be told, they would need help with the mechanics and sometimes the creative interpretation of the story would require a one-on-one arrangement and this is a labor intensive task that requires more than casual commitment of time and caring involvement.

Thirdly, of course, one must work within a structure such as a Day Care Center, a Nursing Home, an Extended Care Center or Retirement Center where groups of frail older adults live and where instruction and assistance can be provided in a relatively direct, inexpensive way. Powhatan Nursing Center and Countryside Manor served as the locations and the instruction was provided on volunteer basis by the author and by students in a Master's degree program. The narrative that follows will show a step-by-step account of the process of beginning an instructional program and the involvement of the University students in producing the short stories that are the focus of the book.

GETTING READY TO SEW (OR WRITE)

A simple diary of events is useful as a guide for reviewing the procedures that lead to the achievement of a goal. It allows others who are interested in working with older adults to repeat the successful portions of the process and to avoid the hazardous or unsuccessful ones. A beginning section of the author's diary follows:

Feb. 5
On February 5th I made a phone call to Powhatan Nursing Center and to Madison Day Care Center to arrange a meeting with the Social Activities director. An appointment was set up for Thursday at 10:00 a.m. to meet with Chris Douglas, Social Activities Director, at Powhatan.

Feb. 13
The appointment with Powhatan people was very interesting. They are anxious to have an educational program. I told them what I had done in nursing centers over the past eight years. They then asked me to come and share these ideas with the staff. Chris (who is super nice) also gave me several hand-outs showing the activities they carry out with patients now. The wheel chair square dancing looks like fun.

Feb. 18
Gave my secretary a copy of the Mental Status Test, Interest Inventory, and a typical lesson plan to reproduce 12 copies of each for sharing with the staff at the meeting on Thursday.

Feb. 20 ·
Went to Powhatan for a session with the staff. Volunteers, music director, and activities director attended (10 in all). I showed them the book, *Teaching and Loving the Elderly* (1983), and gave them the materials the secretary had run off. There are two poems in the book. I read "Is That What You See?" to begin the presentation. I explained the lesson procedure and the reason for the Mental Status Test and for grouping the elderly in different groups to better meet their learning needs. The poem "Gray Courage" was the finale. Questions and answers followed and a copy of the book was left with the staff so that they could make xerox copies of the geragogy

model. It was agreed that the first actual lesson would be on March 20th because the Activities Director and others had a conference for nursing center personnel in Silver Spring, Maryland on March 13th, and so there would not be anyone to help set up the first lesson before then. We all wanted the first lesson to be especially good and to go well.

Feb. 27.

Had to be at the Junior School before 11:00 today to examine the materials there. They have a few good filmstrips which we can use and a limited number of books. Carol (Pyke), the librarian, is great She has an excellent background and much experience and, best of all, she is interested in the program. She will be happy to help me locate materials. I borrowed booklets for Kingdom of Animals and will start making lesson plans right away. Must make the plans enough ahead of time so we can get copies for the "responsible adults" who attend.

March 4

Called Wendy Rogers (Assistant Director, Educational Services) at National Geographic Society on 17th St. in Washington D.C. Asked for free materials for the program — some additional materials are going to be needed if we provide stimulating instructional situations that evoke stories and get the participants fully involved. She was professional, but did not initially volunteer any help (just what I expected). I kept her talking and she agreed to send me their catalogs and then talk some more. She asked if she could attend a session. I said, "Yes, of course!" Maybe we'll get some help. Wouldn't that be wonderful!

March 5

Told Victor Indrisano (Ph.D., Psychology) about the program. He'd like to develop a questionnaire to give to the "responsible adults" who visit the program. Would love to have this as one beginning psychological measure of program effectiveness.

March 11

Have developed the lesson plan but am going to need more information on the buffalo for roomwork reading and questions. Will also need a good map of the U.S. on transparency to show the concentration of animals.

March 12
Victor has a rough draft of the survey form. It looks good. He is going to share it with Chris (Douglas) and Kristin (Colligan), Director of Volunteers, for their comments.

March 18
Went to Powhatan. Had enlargements of the puzzle made, also an enlargement of the buffalo script and the questions to go with it. Robbie Deardon helped with this part of the program. She is going to be a great help — she's a worker bee. She is making copies for the patients. Chris has sent 150 letters to all "responsible adults" asking if they wish to come to the sessions. They have many returns. These gals are SUPER! I get such an emotional boost when I talk with them. They have talked to one woman who has multiple sclerosis. She does not normally go to any of the activities. She doesn't leave her room. Her husband is coming and she initiated making arrangements with the physical therapist to rearrange her time so she can come to the sessions. One minor victory already!

Just got back from the Junior School where I checked out the filmstrip/tape materials. Carol also had 3 books of large print on the topic. The secretary has ordered the filmstrip/tape recorder from the audio-visual lab. We're getting in gear. Chris and Kristin came to see Victor and are all set to run the questionnaire. Cooperation like this is hard to find, and it is so very much needed.

March 18
The filmstrip/tape recorder is an antique. I only hope it works. Now I've tried it and the pictures are clear and good. We'll use up to frame 81 of the filmstrip. Eighty-one frames require a long running time. This is too long for the attention span of the average elderly person. I've certainly run across this problem before. I'm taking a spare overhead bulb in case the one in the machine burns out. I want to ensure the delivery of the lesson.

March 19
Finally, our first lesson! It was a most unbelievable morning, 67 elderly, 14 "responsible adults", 7 people from Madison Day Care

Center, 10-12 staff including the administrator, Mr. Brewster, the assistant administrator, etc., etc. The room was FULL! There was a Proctor & Gamble woman there to give a prize to the Nursing Center for innovative programs and their use of volunteers. This was done before the program started. Then, the lesson began. There was only one plug-in—we needed four in all. The cart the overhead and filmstrip projector were on was narrow and this made it hard to manage the materials. The felt-tipped pen kept rolling off the cart, and the tape wasn't loud enough for such a large room, We got another recorder/player, a blockbuster, to help. BUT, the pictures were beautiful, the spirit was warm and wonderful, and the elderly people enjoyed it greatly. I was so frustrated by media problems that I was completely exhausted afterward. However, if these frail people had an enjoyable learning time, I'm happy. One woman (95 years of age) said, "This has awakened so many thoughts in me. I feel so. . . I guess the word is intellectual." That's what really counts! We'll solve the plug-in/table problems, and the administration is going to have the Great Room wired for special loud speaker systems. This kind of cooperation is impressive.

We (Administrators, Activities personnel and I) did a brief evaluation after the session and are already working on solutions. They will make enlargements of the materials for next week's lessons which I have already planned. I gave them the handouts before I left Powhatan. Wrote a letter to Wendy Rogers. Will call her again Monday.

March 21
I'm working on lesson plans again. It never ends.

March 24
I've gotten the lesson plans and typing of hand-outs to the secretary. Want to get a couple of weeks ahead, if possible.

March 25
Dashed over to Powhatan with the roomwork assignments that needed to be enlarged and the Mental Status collection sheets. We will use these in a week or two. We must separate the group. It is much too large for effective communication or any individual help whatever.

March 27
Just got back from Lesson #2. We had 64 elderly from the Center, 12 "responsible adults," 7 and the Social Activities Director from Madison, and various and sundry personnel from Powhatan. The response was phenomenal! We had elderly people reading the "Who Am I" question sheets — participating in answering questions; much involvement. Malcolm Knowles says that if adults continue to come to the lessons, then, the sessions are a success. Since they are not required to come, they must be enjoying the learning experience. I believe my friend Malcolm is right and I am very pleased with everything so far. The administrators at the Center had a clip-on mike for me and a multiple plug outlet. Really was just super!
Next week it's African wildlife and they are planning to video the entire lesson. It's exciting.

April 1
Gave the materials for next week's lesson to the Social Activities Director who was over here at Marymount to see Victor about his questionnaire. She will take these pages in to be enlarged and this will save me a trip.

April 3
We have just had a really good lesson. There were 67 elderly, 7 from Madison, 12 "responsible adults," 2 great grandchildren (boys ages 6 and 8), plus many staff helpers, as usual. The great grandchildren even helped with the puzzle that was shown on the overhead. Everyone loved the filmstrip, stories and songs. They liked the songs "Kum Ba Yah" and "The Zulu Warrior." The great grandchildren were completely caught up in the lesson and their great grandfather was therefore caught up in the fun.
Contacted National Geographic again today. Have called several times. Put in an order for films, filmstrips, books and maps. They will call back — have been most generous.
Called Dr. Bud Waters (Director of Sponsored Programs at Marymount) and asked him to pursue the FIPSE funding source also.

The diary sequence has been given to provide a little background on the involvement and the planning that is necessary to create a program that is stimulating for the frail older adults for whom it was designed.

NEEDED: A QUILTING BEE

The next problem involved getting helpers who could assist in recording stories and who would respond positively to the elderly people. Elderly people are an important resource for our community and they are collectively one of the elements that has shaped family life for the children in the schools today. Even though this is true, some members of the younger generations may not respond well to them. It was important to have people help record the stories of the elderly and it seemed appropriate that people who plan to teach children in school learn to work with all levels of learners. One course in the education graduate program at Marymount University deals with understanding the community, its needs and its resources. It was a course that the author taught. Graduate students who are preparing to teach in the schools in our communities need to become familiar with the population of elderly folks. Why not have them become acquainted with Powhatan Nursing Center, its programs and the frail older adults who live there? This experience could help prospective teachers become acquainted with the needs of elderly people and the responsibilities that must often be assumed by families in the community to provide adequate care and a quality of life for their older relatives.

Students in the graduate program at Marymount are mature people who are returning to the university following some time spent in another career. They have decided that they wish to teach, but come from different backgrounds and have a wide range of interests. It will be valuable for them to explore several facets of community life. Therefore, five options for field experience are given them in class syllabus. The students are required to select two of the options that follow:

1. Visit two museums and hand in an organized summary statement (no more than 2 pages per museum visit). This should state what you saw and how this might be used with children; approximate grade level should be indicated.

2. Participate in a one night 6-9 p.m. "ride-along" in the Washington D.C. or Arlington, VA, police care "ride along" program. Report this in a brief (2-3 page) written summary.
3. Attend one class at Powhatan Nursing Center as an observer. Then, plan and teach one lesson to the group of frail elderly. The lesson plan will serve as the evaluation base.
4. Visit a local library and make an annotated bibliography of 20 children's books and 10 non-book sources of information at the library. Select a topic and grade level for the development of these materials. Hand in the completed bibliography.
5. Contact the professor about specific tasks for the Department of Human Services in Arlington. Donate 10 hours of time to one of these service areas. Write a 2 page summary of your involvement.

Note that while a range of options is provided for the students, all of the experiences are intended to get them out into the community. The community is a rich resource and the range of resources and human needs can be seen once one gets directly involved in the service areas in the community.

There were 34 students in this class and 8 of them chose to go to the nursing center as one of their options. They observed the author as she developed learning sessions with the group and, then each one of them provided a session for the group of elderly people. The learning experiences the students produced were marvelous! They ranged from learning sessions on Japanese Dolls, to Square Dancing, to a Dog Show, to a session on Puerto Rico. A sample lesson plan from the session on Japanese Dolls follows:

Sample Lesson

Wendy U. Campbell
Lesson Plan: Tuesday, 10:30 a.m.
Powhatan Nursing Home, McLean, VA

A. *Purpose of Lesson:*
This lesson will cover briefly the special significance of the doll in Japanese culture with particular reference to the holiday held on March 3rd known as Girl's Day or Doll's Day.

B. *Behavioral Objective:*
1. While listening to the opening remarks, the students will listen to a Japanese Record.
2. While being given general information about dolls in Japan, the students will observe and touch some dolls of "Old Man" and "Old Woman" significant to Japanese culture.
3. While being given information about the celebration of Doll's Day in Japan, the students will observe the construction of a typical Doll's Day Display and taste (as appropriate) some typical Japanese treats.

C. *Opener:*
The students will listen to a recording of Japanese Bon Odori music: "The Coal Miner's Dance," They will participate in wheelchair version of the dance.

D. *Learning Activities:*
1. The significance of "Old Man" and "Old Woman" in Japanese culture will be explained while the assistants take some examples around for the class to see closely, hold and touch.
2. Observing the construction of the Doll's Day Display and participating in the "tea party" will provide a small introduction to the culture of Japan.

E. *Summary*:
Dolls are significant to every culture. They show a side of the people of that culture which is sometimes difficult to see otherwise. The class will see, hear, touch, and taste a little bit of Japan.

F. *Evaluation*:
Evaluation will be based on the level of participation shown through interest, questions, and enthusiasm.

G. *Materials*:
Doll's Day Set-Up: Emperor & Empress, Ladies, Musicians, Councilor, Furniture, Red Cloth
"Old Man" and "Old Woman" Dolls: porcelain, kime-kome, little set of happy pair
Tray, plates, Doll's Day candles, and crackers
Record Player and Record: "The Coal Miner's Dance"

Other students also directed sessions in which they asked the older participants to produce ideas, and to talk about parts of the session that interested them. They then asked participants if any of them had ever been to Japan, had owned dogs, had enjoyed square dancing, and so forth. The students asked the elderly participants to tell about these experiences. The students who attended the sessions were fascinated by the stories that the older folks told.

Finally one of the students, Nan Cooper, brought in a display of patchwork quilts and encouraged the participants to talk about them. One woman said that these patchwork quilts were like the group, a lot of people from different backgrounds who had a lot of old fashioned memories. A book idea was born! A patchwork of memories, sure enough!

LEARNING TO USE THIMBLES

Learning experiences were presented for several weeks to pre-pare the older folks to tell stories that could be shared with other people. The need for each elderly person to write about their life's experiences was stressed. Several topics were presented to prepare the group to write. The writing of myths and what they represent was perhaps the first topic explored by the group. A myth is a tradi-tional story about an event or an occurrence, and it serves to explain people, events, beliefs or a natural phenomenon. Several Indian myths were read to the group and an echo play based on the book THE FIRE BRINGER, A Paiute Indian Legend (1972), was en-acted by the group. Participants took part with enthusiasm and de-veloped costumes that could be used even as they acted out their parts from wheelchairs. Finally, the group was asked to produce a myth of their own. The following is an example of a myth they produced:

HOW SUNSETS BECAME RED

The sky was blue during the day and as evening came, the sun began to set in the West. The gods did not wish to see the sun disappear and they were angry. They were angry, too, because all the people were fighting for land. The gods thought the people were being greedy. They sought revenge, and although they could not prevent the sun from setting, they changed it into a ball of fire as it went down. The whole sky reflected the brilliant flames of the sun. To this day whenever people become greedy, the sun again turns to flame and, the sunset is red and threatening. The gods are angry again and we see their anger in the fire of the sun.

A lesson on how to make appropriate illustrations for a story was provided and the elderly were encouraged to illustrate the myth. The suggestions for illustrations particularly interested one woman who was herself an artist. Others had been good at sketching and they enjoyed the ideas about illustration. Overhead materials were used to give order to developing illustrations. The following transparencies were shown and discussed in some detail using examples from books:

Transparency #1 – Objectives of illustration

IN GENERAL AN ILLUSTRATION SHOULD:
1. Fulfill its function
    a. point out a particular character
    b. sell a product
    c. focus on a significant idea
2. Be attractive
3. Appeal to an identifiable audience

Transparency #2 – Methods of illustrating

METHODS FOR ACHIEVING OBJECTIVES
IN ILLUSTRATING

I. MAKE A CENTRAL THEME STAND OUT
    A. Contrast in hue
        1. Light and dark
        2. Black and white
    B. Complex areas against simplified ones
    C. Control the design by using insets
    D. Control the design by using open spaces

II. MAKE ONLY ONE FIGURE OR DESIGN
Use abstract or other non-traditional design

III. MATCH THE THEME
A. Use cultural art
B. Use objects that are natural

In separate lessons, we covered topics dealing with writing stories about historic events, adventure stories and life's experiences. The elderly were given roomwork with each of these assignments and were gradually being prepared to write stories on their own. Some of the detail for each of these sessions will be presented as the stories are given in the book.

Now, with the aid of the students it was possible to record the stories the elderly could tell and a simple review of the lesson ideas was all that was needed. We talked again about adventure stories, stories of historical events, and the way in which life experiences might be recorded. Students worked for several weeks recording ideas, then writing them up in story form; taking them back and checking for accuracy and redoing them. The elder who told the story was shown the final product and his/her approval was sought. Some persons pondered the title of their stories for a long time; they wished to have it catch the eye of the reader. Probably, about eight weeks of time was needed to accumulate the stories and to polish them. The students thoroughly enjoyed the interaction with the elders and there were many comments from the older adults showing clearly that they enjoyed the chance to talk with an interested younger person. The following materials include the preparation for building up ideas about adventure stories, for example, and the actual adventure stories themselves.

Chapter II

The Quilting Process

Preparation is a major factor in quilting and it is in writing stories, as well. This is true for any writer whatever the age of the individual. It is important for older adults and is perhaps even more necessary for very old people because they need time to think about and organize the details of the events they wish to describe. A number of lessons were provided to prepare the elderly participants with the opportunity to verbalize. In a survey with two other nursing center groups it was determined that elderly people enjoy learning about early America or colonial days (see John, 1983). A series of lessons was designed on this topic and discussion was planned for each of the lessons. It is important to get the participant talking freely and generating ideas as they speak. Some have been living alone prior to coming to the nursing center and communication has been minimal. Here is an example of one of the lesson plans used and a sample team role playing exercise the elderly participated in as a part of the session.

ROOM ARRANGEMENT

One of the things that the volunteer must consider before actually presenting the mental stimulation session is the physical arrangement of the room. It is important that the participants be placed in comfort and that they be in a position to see the overhead materials and the opening media presentation. Several options exist for room arrangement. Here are two different ones (see Option I). There are any number of other alternatives.

The designs presented are based on the idea that there will be small numbers of people and that there will be tables available for

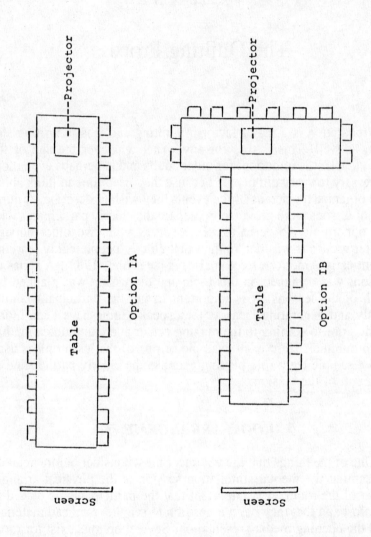

them to use in the class session. The following example is one that can be used when there are a large number of participants and it does not require tables (see Option II). However, because there are no tables, there can be no written response required of the participants as the instruction goes forward.

ACTUAL INSTRUCTIONAL SESSION

One of the primary objectives of the instructional sessions was to get these frail elderly people to respond to new learning experiences. This might require a verbal or a non-verbal response, but the use of language was a vital part of the expected reaction. To that end a number of special stimulation techniques were used.

Mental Stimulation

Instructional Session: "America: Colonization to Constitution"

Specific Materials: Filmstrip, "Years of War: Lexington to Valley Forge"; filmstrip and tape from the National Geographic Society; overhead of—vocabulary, discussion questions, "Yankee Doodle." Handouts of loyalist and patriot, "Paul Revere's Ride" and roomwork.

Purpose: To help particpants review the struggle that helped our country begin, and to use new ideas as they are presented.

1. Given a list of vocabulary words, the participants will review their meaning prior to viewing the filmstrip.
2. Given a filmstrip/tape presentation the participants will attend.
3. Given the poem "Paul Revere's Ride," the participants will do a choral reading of it.
4. Given a series of questions, the participants will verbally discuss the issues these involve.
5. Given a team role playing situation between a loyalist and a patriot, the participants will all take part in the dilemma.
6. Given an opportunity to sing "Yankee Doodle," the participants will participate.
7. Given roomwork, the particpants will complete the work within the following week.

Procedure

Opener: What would you think if I told you that Paul Revere was one of the first members of our intelliegence service? What role did this play in the results of the Revolutionary War?

Learning Experiences: The participants will:

1. Read the terms and the definitions of the following words:

artillery	courier	Minutemen
musket	outflank	patriot

2. View the filmstrip.
3. Read "Paul Revere's Ride" in a choral fashion.
4. Discuss:
   1. What do you think of when you hear the word "revolution"?
   2. Would you approve of a "Boston Tea Party" today?
   3. What do you think "the shot heard round the world" means?
   4. Could the phrase, "These are the times that try men's souls," be used today.
   5. What would it mean today?

5. Participate in a team role playing session involving descriptions of loyalists and partiots. (See Sample I for role-playing sequence.)
6. Sing "Yankee Doodle."
7. Receive roomwork.

Summary and Futuristic challenge: Verbal summary and the idea of Places Where Plants and Animals Live will be stressed as a colorful new topic.

Evaluation:

1. Note correct number of responses.
2. Note the participation in the role playing and singing.

Materials: Filmstrip, tape, overhead and transparencies for it, poem, song and role playing descriptions, roomwork.

*Note: For the role playing session, it might be wise to arrange
participants in small groups around tables for better interaction. See Figure 1 for a sample arrangement.

On Learning Experience 5 there is the mention of a role-playing
session. One way to help groups of people identify the feelings
involved in any decision making process is role-playing. Here is an
example of the materials that were prepared for the session men-
tioned in learning experience number 5.

Task Instructions:

1. Have two slips of paper prepared with a description of a person on each piece of paper.
2. Do not read the descriptions aloud. Tell participants that they
   shoud not read the descriptions to each other. The descriptions
   should be kept secret for the time being.
3. Hand out descriptions.
4. Tell participants that they are all allowed to speak at the same
   time.
5. They should be prepared to answer the question, "Why do I
   want independence?".
6. Use a vignette like the following:

Sample I:
Team Role Play

1. You have lived in the New World for several years. You su-
pervise your family's shipping business in America. You are realiz-
ing good profits and look forward to retiring comfortably on the
family property in England. During your stay here, you have had to
travel a lot and are aware of the unrest in the colonies. You believe
most of the colonists were malcontents to begin with, and many
were "transported" from their native country on criminal charges
or left England to escape bankruptcy. You've met a lot of rough
characters who seem to prove it. Still, you deal with them as honor-
ably as you can and you are careful to trade fairly. You miss London and genteel English society. You're proud to be called a Tory
and a King's man, and you keep company with other Tory families

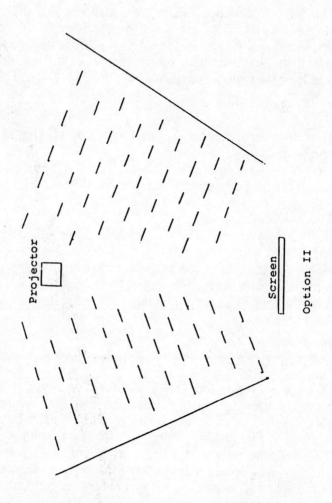

Projector

Screen

Option II

FIGURE 1

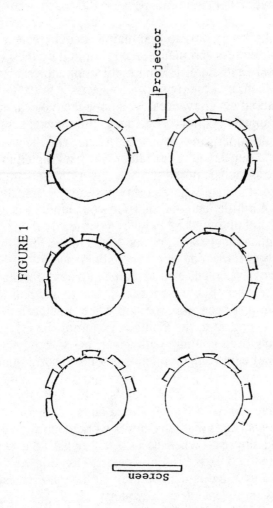

who preserve English tastes and manners—music, dancing, elegant dress and housekeeping. Tonight, however, you've had to interrupt a journey between shipping ports because the coach needed repairs. You've taken a room at an inn. You're hungry after your day and enter the smoky tavern only to find that the people there are not too happy with your dress and manner. You can tell by their conversation that they are anti-English. You don't want unpleasantness, and when one of them makes a remark about you, you try to talk with him directly about his grievances. You hope that you can make him see that the "injustices" he complains about are exaggerated.

2. You are an American colonist, born here, and the word "colonist" sticks in your throat. Your father was bankrupted in England and came here as an indentured servant, a working servant, working seven years for the man who paid his passage. Eventually he was able to acquire a little land and married your mother. This is your country and you fail to understand why your legal affairs should be settled by English magistrates, or taxes paid to the English at a rate you can barely afford. You don't feel allegiance to the King of a country you've never seen. You've come into town for market day, not just to do business but to meet friends and to talk politics. Some new laws have just been imposed and when a delegation of land-owners went to protest to the Colonial governor, he refused to see them. You have been seething with anger, but you are also a God-fearing man and believe that violence is a last resort. Nonetheless, people are talking about taking up arms against the English. You wonder if you should listen. Now there's an English fat-cat drinking in the town tavern next to you. It's hard not to drop a few remarks when you see his hands that have never worked hard, as you have. You're a little surprised when he asks you what your complaints are. Does he really not know? You decide to tell him what it is like to be governed by a Parliament where you have no representative. "'Why do I want independence?' you say . . . "

SAMPLE I

Next Week: From this point the teacher proceeded to a session on "Farm Life" in colonial days and folks discussed all sorts of itmes, like plows, harrows, oxen, grain cradles, windrows; what winnowing and broadcasting meant, and finally what farms were like when they were young.

The next lesson presented a filmstrip/tape on "crafts" in pioneer days and the questions the participants responded to were like the following:

1. Have you ever worked a spinning wheel?
2. What is the sequence used in making a sweater from fleece to the finished product? (carding, combing, spinning, winding into skeins, twisting and knotting, knitting and, finally piecing together)
3. Have you ever seen or worked a loom?
4. What is the method by which a loom weaves cloth?
5. What materials can be used to make braided rugs? (old clothes, new wool)
6. What is the fabric base for a hooked rug? (burlap)
7. What examples of men's crafts were shown? (carving an axe handle, making farm tools, and designing leather for harnesses)
8. What two different types of candles were shown? (dipped, molded)
9. Are any of the crafts practiced by the pioneers used today?
10. Which craft might be most useful today? Why?

The teacher or the individual preparing the group for writing exercises may wish to personalize an event or an idea that is being studied. This will give the older student a better chance to relate to the idea in a direct way. One way to do this is to go to each person with a microphone and request information such as the place she/he was born or the family name, for example. One could then apply this information to a specific geography lesson or to the origin of names in the New World. Frequently, the personalization of information is dependent upon the skill of the teacher and it may be a spur of the moment response to some comment from one of the participants. The teacher may note a special interest or hear an answer to a question that makes the eyes of the listeners light up. The time to pursue the idea has come when this happens.

A number of other exercises have been used to stimulate the development and use of vocabulary in preparation to the writing exercises that are the ultimate goal of these sessions. In one series of instructional sessions, for example, the participants were taken for a "Travel Log" experience and a number of foreign countries were presented. Roomwork activities were provided for each of the countries and one of the ones for Great Britain was an assignment where the participants were to write as many words as possible from the name of one of the cathedrals. They had seen beautiful slides of the cathedral as part of the instructional input. One of the participants came back the next week with the list shown in Figure 2.

An actual copy of the work done by the particpant is given so that the reader can see the work and thinking of the writer.

FIGURE 2

WINCHESTER CATHEDRAL

win	earl	the	nail	little	was	start
chest	this	he	tail	whittle	saw	area
Hester	China	Eric	its	Rath	with	hair
cat	as	darn	dice	awe	here	wren
Edna	later	alert	lice	dance	dan	reward
her	herd	are	nice	while	can	ward
dart	wind	white	rice	street	hand	chart
Pleiadeswinter	Santa	wise	Kansas	Randell	shard
Helen	west	distaste	dial	retire	sand	snarl
Ina	watched	ana	sin	learned	Wanda	nest
Dana	wart	and	din	district	Chester	stir
head	water	herd	hind	Easter	watt	rind
heat	whirl	seated	liner	dress	rest	wench
hat	wet	what	rhine	sale	least	wrench
heart	lard	scared	sinew	classic	red	drawl
had	let	ladies	tines	Clara	dear	card
has	last	care	thin	steel	deer	hard
hail	when	dare	then	ends	cheer	girl
mind	rise	hare	hen	estate	tend	swirl
cast	tend	leer	at	star	can	in
cane	sir	near	lend	water	tear	are
is	new	wear	send	rend	dreary	rain
his	wear	rear	wend	wares	wheat	lair
handel	care	tale	twin	Danish	can	than
dale	hale	late	rear	hatter	chatter	shirt
ear	lane	cane	rain	cain	den	there
cart	nearer	dearest

For additional samples of ideas that have been used with success to stimulate the thinking of the elderly population, see Appendix A.

EXAMINING PATTERNS

One of the elements in preparation for writing is practice in writing. For many of our elderly folks it may have been a long time since they wrote about happenings in their lives. Some had never done so. Practice sessions utilized list poems and sentence completing like: "I remember the first day I ever went to school, I . . . . " and "The first train ride my family went on was when . . . ."Other similar open-ended sentences were used and as many as possible were asked to respond into the microphone so that others could share their memories. After all, that was what our writing was all about.

Here is a sample of one of the color poems the group composed.

Green

Green is the color of grass
Green is the color of leaves, but they won't last,
Green goes with red at Christmas time,
Green is the color of a holiday rhyme
Green is the beginning of spring
Green is the color of a cheap ring.
Green is the emerald of seasons,
Green is good for any reason.
Eyes are green, envy is too;
After a storm, green skies turn to blue
Green is clean, it's a natural hue.
Green is a color that makes me rest,
Green is the color that I like best.

EXAMINING DIFFERENT BLOCKS

Before any actual writing or even any dictation takes place, it is wise to provide specific instruction about the writing process in which the folks are about to participate. Practice sessions may be needed to deal with the organization of ideas, the elaboration of ideas, the use of primary and secondary sources of information, and being able to tell the difference between fact and opinion. All of these elements can enter into the stories they are about to write and may influence the degree to which other people can enjoy their stories to the fullest.

Here is a sample worksheet, on "Fact and Opinion" that the elderly participants at Powhatan responded to.

FACT VS. OPINION

FACT: A statement which can be shown with actual evidence to be true.

OPINION: A judgement or view held by one or more individual, often unsupported by facts.

In order to determine whether a statement is fact or opinion, ask yourself the following questions:

1. Can the statement be proven? (fact)
2. Is the statement repeating someone's ideas about something? (opinion)

The sentence, "The Battle of Hastings took place in 1066," is a statement of fact since there is documented evidence supporting it. The sentence, "Nestles makes the very best chocolate," is a statement of opinion since not everyone would agree that it is true.

DIRECTIONS: Write Fact or Opinion in front of each statement below.

_____ 1. *GONE WITH THE WIND* is the best movie ever made.
_____ 2. *GONE WITH THE WIND* won many Academy Awards.
_____ 3. Jimmy Stewart was a better actor than Jimmy Cagney.
_____ 4. P.B.S. shows many programs made for B.B.C.
_____ 5. The B.B.C. programs are the best programs on TV today.
_____ 6. Masterpiece Theater has been on every Sunday night for more than 10 years.
_____ 7. It is better to go to the movies than to watch television.
_____ 8. Everybody loves going to the theater.
_____ 9. *The Washington Post* publishes a weekly TV guide with its Sunday paper.

_____ 10. TV is a waste of time.

_____ 11. Public television stations run very few commercials.

_____ 12. The play, *Les Miserables*, won a Tony Award in 1987.

COLORFUL PHRASES

A discussion about creative stories was part of the preparation for writing. Participants were given a number of exercises like the following one. These were shared on a transparency and the suggestions of several people were incorporated into the finished sentences

Adjectives and adverbs lend color to dull sentences. No one would want to read stories like this one.

> "I went for a walk. It was cold. There were many cars. There were many people, too. I came back home."

Color could be added to this story by elaborating on the story and using adjectives and adverbs in the right places. Here are several dull sentences. Participants at the Nursing Home were told to add color by using two descriptors in the sentences. This is a sample of one man's work.

1. The dog ran down the street.
   Rewrite: The German Shepherd loped gracefully down the shady lane.
2. The man ate his meal.
   Rewrite: The emaciated man ate the vegetable beef stew ravenously.
3. The night was long.
   Rewrite: The rustling of night creatures in the surrounding bushes and the hooting of the owls in the deep forest added to our fears and made the moonless night seem endless.
4. The farmer went to the market.
   Rewrite: The industrious farmer carried his finest produce to market at 6 a.m. on Saturdays to catch the discriminating early shoppers.
5. The ground was wet with dew.
   Rewrite: Early morning dew sparkled on spider webs like diamonds and freshly washed each blade of grass.

REVIEW ACTION IDEAS

It is useful to review ideas about the action, conflict and suspense that one expects to find in an adventure story. Adventures have happened to everyone and it really boils down to the telling of the tale that makes it exciting and spine tingling for the listener. There are some general "rule-of-thumb" ideas to remember in writing an adventure story. Since adventure stories convey action, conflict and suspense, it is important to keep verbs in mind. Verbs convey action! Exercises emphasizing verb choices were designed and used with the folks at Powhatan to encourage them to consider different ways of expressing conflict or suspense. Here are a few examples of the exercises used.

Adventure (Pupil Follow-Up)

Action, Conflict, and Suspense

DIRECTIONS: Answer True or False to the following statements:

_____ 1. This sentence contains *suspense*:
The boy's eyes widened as the gigantic cobra raised its head only inches from his own.

_____ 2. This sentence suggests *action*:
The crowd cheered as the horses rounded the turn with the Big Black in the lead by a nose.

_____ 3. This sentence suggests *conflict*:
The three little kittens quietly lapped up their milk.

Writing with Action Words

DIRECTIONS: Choose the word that will achieve the most action-filled sentence.

1. A scream _____ through the night.
   sounded, tore
2. The children _____ down the road.
   went, raced
3. The fear _____ up and _____ the scream in her throat.
   welled, came   strangled, kept

4. The rocks _____ down the hill.
   hurtled, rolled
5. A stranger _____ into the room.
   walked, strode boldly

Using Title Cards

DIRECTIONS: In which card catalogue drawer would you find the following title cards?

_____ 1. *Robin Hood*
_____ 2. *The Sword in the Stone*
_____ 3. *A Tale Of Two Cities*
_____ 4. *Mr. Chips*

A STITCH IN TIME

Elderly people enjoy remembering past experiences, particularly ones from long ago when their world was quite different. Often grandchildren will beg granddad or grandma for a story about when they were young. The grandchild frequently cannot quite believe that the story is altogether true. Who could imagine a world without television, without cars, without electric lights or other modern conveniences? The stories sometimes take on the flavor of fairy tales and perhaps this is one of the reasons the grandchildren are so fascinated with them.

Since many of the people in the nursing home were confined physically, many in wheelchairs or wheelbeds, it is not surprising that they liked thinking about situations in which they could run about as free as the breeze. We talked about past times and materials such as filmstrips, pictures and worksheets about early America were developed with teacher guidance. The focus was on historical events; things that happened within their lifetime, but very long ago. Here are some examples of the materials used with the participants at Powhatan Nursing Center to prepare them for writing or dictating their story about historical events.

A filmstrip/tape about Historical Fiction (Pied Piper Productions) was used to help stimulate thinking about historic events in which elderly participants might have been involved. This was followed by a discussion which reviewed the events that have taken place since they were born. Several of the individuals present had been born before 1900, and could remember many details about World War I and the Great Depression. We explored these memories in some detail as a group. Sometimes questions arose about a particular event and there seemed to be some question about the actual sequence of events or perhaps the accuracy of the remembrance of it. Then, the idea of using other sources of information to verify the accuracy of the sequence was proposed.

An overhead transparency was used to collect the responses of the group and a list of the places one could use to verify a story was developed by the participants.

Primary Sources of Information

1. People
2. Your own experience
3. Police records
4. Newspapers (at the time of the event)
5. Letters
6. Diaries
7. Archives
8. Old photographs
9. Scrapbooks
10. Land grant records
11. Assessor's books
12. Wills
13. Family Bibles
14. Family account books

Note how much more creative the group became as they progressed from number one to number fourteen. Actually, the list is quite comprehensive.

Following this exercise, the participants were given two peices of roomwork which dealt with primary and secondary sources of information.

Historical Fiction

DIRECTION: Answer True or False to the following statements.

_____1. Historical fiction is often based upon researched facts.

_____2. All historical fiction is about kings and queens.

_____3. In a library you would find historical fiction in the history section.

_____4. The following sentence is an example of imagination blended with historical fact: The Big Bad Wolf huffed and he puffed, 'til he blew the house down.

Research for Historical Fiction

DIRECTIONS: Complete the answer by matching the left column with the right column.

1. To personally experience how a character might have lived.
2. To find the distance.
3. To see the Hope Diamond.
4. To gather several opinions on a subject.
5. To get a first-hand experience of Paris.

a. Consult several sources.
b. Visit a museum.
c. Use a map or atlas.
d. Read a primary source.
e. Personally visit places of interest to the plot or character.

ARE WE READY?

The background information has been given. Hopefully, the reader has seen that preparing for the writing task is not a simple one. The cooperation of the volunteer staff at the nursing center was required. (Who brings all the persons needing assistance to the Commons Room for the sessions? Why, the volunteers and the social activitees directors, of course.)

The students from Marymount University were needed to record the stories, to rewrite them after jotting down or tape recording the ideas from the elderly person with whom they worked. The teacher or group leader was required to carry out administrative tasks and prepare learning sessions. In these sessions, practice in verbalizing about happenings in their lives, thinking about myths, adventures, historic events and life's experiences was necessary. Finally, the stories are ready for the participants of Powhatan Nursing Center to share.

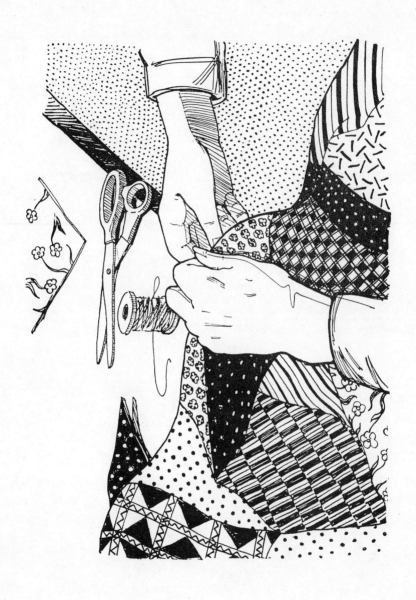

Chapter III

Antique Quilt Pieces
(Historical Stories)

The folks at Powhatan told some stories that had interesting bits of history in the telling. For instance, the story Elsie Marvin tells about dancing with a Civil War veteran is rather unique. You will enjoy these short stories about happenings some 80 or more years ago.

THE DANCE OF A LIFETIME

I danced with a Civil War Veteran! It was the Virginia Reel. I couldn't have been more than about eight at the time and he was an older person, but so graceful and kind to me. He was dressed in his beautiful, old uniform and everyone watched us as we danced.

We had gone to the Relief Corps Dance and they had a sentry at the door, very tall and stately. My mother belonged to the Relief Corps, a kind of women's auxiliary. They had lots of programs, you know, Christmas and Santa Claus, that sort of thing. That was our society life, going to the Relief Corps meeting. But, I'd never danced with a Vet before.

My Grandfather had been in the Civil War, but he had not fought. They sent him home with the measles, of all things! I loved my Grandfather dearly. He used to walk to my house daily and always had peppermints in his pocket. We'd play casino, just him and me. He finally became a judge in Berkeley, California, and enjoyed sharing his stories of his short war experiences with his friends.

I grew up in Berkeley and raised a family there of my own. My daughter graduated from the University of California at Berkeley in 1962 and became a teacher.

My husband worked for Remington Rand for 40 years out there. He graduated from Chino State Normal School in 1915 and tried to be a teacher, but Remington Rand paid better. After he retired, he grew pretty restless. My daughter said, "Dad, there's an older man with red hair who subs at my school. The kids just love him." Well, he decided to try it and he was hired right away. He worked as a sub until he was 80 years old. All the kids in the area knew him. The phone would ring every night about dinner time. It would be one of the little boys from school and they'd talk baseball or something. He sure loved that job.

I remember the last time they called. He was so sick but he was considering it, I could tell. So I just shook my head and he told the person on the phone, "My wife says I can't come, I'm sorry," sorta' like you'd say, "My Mom says I can't come out and play now."

After my husband died I came to Virginia to be near my daughter and her family. She has two sons and the grandsons are so much fun. The oldest is off training boys at Boy Scout Camp this year. They're both Scouts and I love them dearly. I don't often have peppermints in my pocket like my Civil War Grandpa did, but I think they love me too.

To this day whenever I hear music like the Virginia Reel, I remember the tall gentleman who was willing to dance with a big-eyed little girl all those years ago. Somehow, the Civil War and the men who had fought in it always seemed more real to me after that one memorable Virginia Reel.

—Elsie Marvin

THE AGE OF INVENTION

I was born in the age of invention,
When things were beginning to change,
And now, friends, it is my intention
To give you a taste of that age.

I was born in the house on 15th Street
It was common enough then, you see.

My mother's uncle was the doctor
Who delivered my sister and me.

The washing machine and the dryer,
the light bulb and first fridgedair
Were things yet to be discovered.
When I first became truly aware.

Before electricity became servants,
To help us with all in our home,
We beat out our rugs, hand washed dishes.
We had gas to bring light to our rooms.

There were mesh caps to put on the burners.
They were fragile and easily torn.
Mother said, "Children, be careful!
They cost one quarter each, so be warned!"

They were quite pretty things, I remember,
As was much which is now different.
The school with the limestone decorations,
Downtown where my free time was spent.

I remember my father in wartime,
And when he came back, we were glad
They sold extra runs of the paper.
THE WAR IS NOW OVER!, it said.

I was born in the age of invention
I've enjoyed watching everything grow.
The changes there've been in my lifetime,
Have been very exciting, you know.

—Elizabeth Sullivan Coulon
As interpreted by Wendy Campbell

THE HOUSE ON 21st STREET IN ARLINGTON

I was 19 years old when I came up here from Tennessee. I was scared to death! It happened I knew some friends who were to meet me at the station and help me to get settled. I was certainly glad to see a friendly face as I stepped from that train, I can tell you.

There it was—The Capital City. It was a pretty small town compared to what it is now, but it was exciting enough to me. I felt quite the lady as they whisked me off to Mrs. Moore's Boarding House.

What can I tell you about Mrs. Moore? She was one of those older women that, you know, nothing ever suited her. She was from Tennessee and felt strongly about that. But I will tell you this — she sure took care of those she liked. There were seven of us staying there at the time. We all ate together in the big dining room and we got to know each other pretty well. Upstairs there were five boys. "Her Boys" she called them: one from Tennessee, one from Kentucky and one from Missouri . . . THOSE BOYS! Mrs. Moore, being from Tennessee herself, took a special liking to me and my roommate, Lucille Peterson. We all took to calling Lucille " Pat " for some reason, and "Pat" and I write to each other to this day.

Well, I began to settle in. I soon found a job working for the Census Bureau and began to step out with a young man from upstairs. I was feeling very grown-up. I had quite decided to go off on my own, but my young man, the man I was to marry, said, "No, Dorothy, you don't need to go off on your own. You take Pat with you." So Pat and I took rooms together until we married.

Once my husband and I were married, we went to live in the little house on 21st street in Arlington. He worked for the Library of Congress, you know. He did something I never quite understood with books. Well, there, on 21st Street is where we brought first Karen and then Philip into the world. It has always seemed to be home to me even though we have lived in many places since.

During World War II, my husband went to serve for two years and once again, didn't want me to be "on my own." So he sent us down to Kentucky to stay with his relatives. It always seemed so useless to me. They didn't know what to do with us, nor we with them . . . they didn't care much for kids, and ours were little then. And we did so miss the house on 21st Street in Arlington.

After the war was over, it didn't take us long to get back in the swing of things. We were among the lucky ones. So many had died, others came home injured and many had to search for jobs and places to live. The Library of Congress had saved my husband's job for him. We had only lost one friend during that whole long fight.

We had our kids, our future and we were home again, back in the little house on 21st Street, in Arlington, Virginia.

— Dorothy Karsner
As told to Wendy Campbell

MEMORIES ON BASEBALL

My favorite game is baseball.
I used to read about baseball games.
Mainly I would read the newspapers.
I would read baseball stories and collector stories.
The teams that I read about are long gone.
My favorite team was the N.Y. Yankees
They wore baggy pants.
Their colors were blue and black.
Babe Ruth was my favorite player.
He was a popular player.
He was a big league hitter.
He struck out many players.

— Dorothy Ryan
As adapted by Kathy Koczyk

A TERRIFYING EXPERIENCE

I was born in Philadelphia and moved to the country when I was seven. A school friend moved down to Washington and invited me to come visit. She and her husband had invited a friend to go fishing. He said that he didn't like to fish, but *would* like to meet a nice girl, so they found just the one for him. When I arrrived they invited him to the house. He took me to a movie and afterwards we sat in the car and talked and talked. When I went inside, they all crowded around and asked me about the date. Later, I went to the beach and my friends talked me into sending a card to him. If my mother had known, she would have wanted me to marry him right then! Those friends could not even go to our wedding because there was a polio epidemic and the town was under quarantine.

I would read baseball stories and collector stories. The teams that I read about are long gone. My favorite game is baseball. I used to read about baseball games. mainly. I would read the newspapers.

He struck out many players. He was a big leaguer. He was a popular man. and Ruth was my favorite. Babe Ruth was. His colors were Blue. N.Y. pants. Their my favorite team was the Yankees. They were Biggy.

My family was Irish Catholic and my father always told us to love one another. I was the oldest of three girls and if we would get angry with each other my grandmother would put us in separate rooms. My mother was a perfect lady. I never heard her yell. My intended's family was very different.

When I went to meet them for the first time, my husband told me not to worry. He said that his father was sulking, but it didn't mean anything. I never heard of a man sulking before. When Mrs. Trapp introduced me to Mr. Trapp, she took me by the hand and said, "This is the little girl our son has been going to see." He never even took my hand.

At the end of the weekend when I met the Trapp family, I was to take the train home on Sunday night. My intended put me on the train and gave the porter some money. He told the porter to "take good care" of me. Well, he certainly did! I had to get off at a certain station to catch a local. It was dark, and when the train stopped, the porter put me off on the mail platform! The train ran high above the town on elevated tracks, and the mail platform was off to the side of the tracks. The station was far below and the only way to get there was to walk down the tracks upon which my train had just disappeared. Fortunately, I was familiar with the town, because I had gone to school there and was friends with people from both sides of the tracks. I could hear people on the street below and knew that I must get someone's attention. I thought they would notice if I dropped my scarf, since they couldn't hear me. Helplessly, I watched the scarf flutter slowly to the ground and fall behind the couple. The next time, I decided to drop something heavier. My gold compact had my name, address, and telephone number marked on the inside. I took it from the pocketbook which I had over my shoulder and waited for someone else to come. Finally I heard voices. When it seemed that they were directly below me, I dropped my precious gold compact. It saved my life, but I never saw it again. Those passerby went to the station for help. I saw the lantern coming up the tracks toward me. An older man — he must have been at least 65 — came to get me. He moved quickly and said, "Now you follow me and don't look down. We have to move fast because the express train from Philadelphia to New York is coming soon."

I missed the local train and had to take the milk run home. My mother hadn't slept at all that night, and wanted to know what had happened, but I never did tell her. She didn't want me to go to work the next day, but I had to go. I didn't know how upset I had been until I tried to type and found that I couldn't because my hands were shaking so hard. I shook every time I thought of it for long time.

—Frances Quinn Trapp
As told to Jan Vincent

OLD BUILDINGS JOG MEMORIES

During the past few days my brother-in-law, Amos, has torn down an old barn on my place. Naturally, I have been much interested in the project as the building was an unsightly old thing and its days of usefulness were over, and it will be a joy to have it down and the spot cleaned up. But there's also a feeling of regret because the tearing down had to be done; a good deal like the feeling you have when you have to discard an old hat, or suit, which has given you good service over a long period of time.

The old barn started its existence as a house and it stood several rods back from the road, across the road and souteast from my house. It was built by late Henry Kent, on land then owned by him, for his daughter and son-in-law, soon after they were married nearly ninety years ago. The house was built of balsam logs and was almost twenty feet square.

Some ten or twelve years after the building of the house, the late Anthony Sprague bought the place where I now live and a little later bought the log house which was then standing vacant, and was said to be haunted. Anthony took the building apart and rebuilt it over here, adding a "lean-to" on the south side of it to house his cattle and horses. The log part was used for hay storage.

In May, 1922, my husband Albert and I bought this place from Mr. Sprague. At the time we owned only one cow and one horse, but we soon began to "farm it," and to clean up the larger fields. It wasn't long before we had the barn full and running over with both stock and hay. From the first Albert bought, raised and sold cattle and I always helped where I could—feeding calves, watering stock, cleaning stables, milking cows—just doing anything I could to help.

Through the years we had several horses and many a time we spent the most of the night doctoring a sick horse or cow. If an animal was sick, Amos always helped us at such times.

Full well I remember the first team that Albert bought after we lived here. They were half-brothers, each nine years old. Bill was bay-colored, calm and even tempered. Cooney was coal black and nervous. In reality, he was kind, too, but he never acted it. Most people were afraid of him because he would tramp and tread and switch his tail, lay back his ears and snap his teeth. You could easily believe he was going to trample you to death, or eat you alive. He had only one thing that he did that was really bad. He would snap at your hand if you did not take the water pail away just the instant he was through drinking. Once he grabbed Albert's cousin on the top of his head instead of on the hand. He tore Ken's cap off and thinned out his hair considerably.

I was really just a little scared of Cooney, but just a year or two after we got the horses, Albert broke his leg one summer and I had to do most of the chores. We sprayed the cattle twice a day to keep the flies from pestering them so, but the horses were afraid of the noise that the sprayer made. Albert had been in the habit of dampening a cloth and wiping it over the horses' faces, necks, breasts, bellies and legs. One day when the flies were especially bad, I decided to rub the fly spray on them the same as Albert did. The horses stood together in a wide stall with only a pole between them. The pole was fastened possibly three feet high at the manger end and rested on the floor at the other end.

I got Bill done alright and was working on Cooney while standing on Bill's side of the pole, and somehow I fell over the pole, and landed on the floor, flat on my back under Cooney's belly. Instantly, the thought came that I would be trampled to death, because every little thing made him so nervous. I called out, "Whoa, Cooney, whoa!" And do you know, I think that horse had no intention of doing anything else but "Whoa," for he stood absolutely still. He didn't even shake his head or switch his tail. I had to turn over and crawl out from under him before I could get up, but still he stood, motionless. When I was on my feet again, he became the same old Cooney as I finished the fly-repellent job. Seeing the old barn torn down made me think of that horse.

Our daughters also have memories connected with the old barn which they will not soon forget. Their most pleasant ones are of the nights about once or twice during each summer, usually when the barn was about two-thirds full of new hay, when their cousins Mary Ellen, Anna, Emma, Katherine, Geneva and Leonora would come over and the girls would each take a blanket or quilt and sleep on the new-mown hay. At least they spent the night there. Such nights were usually filled with visiting, laughing, singing and joking until the wee hours. Probably, there was a bit of sleeping in the early morning hours before they would come in for a big breakfast.

And so the years went by. The old barn was crammed full of memories, some good, some not so good, but always and always the memories had to do with the tasks that Albert and I did together. The old barn HAD to come down, but the memories will remain.

—Helen Escha Tyler

A HEARTBREAKING EXPERIENCE

About seventy years ago, I went to Puerto Rico as a representative of Governor Franklin D. Roosevelt of New York State. Our joint interest was to make a personal survey of the results of a disastrous hurricane which swept across the interior areas of Puerto Rico. This called for a national campaign for assistance to the people of Puerto Rico—medical supplies, food, and clothing.

In this report I shall not go further into my experiences in visiting many of the mountainous areas which bore the brunt of the hurricane. Instead, I want to relate briefly a strange and memorable experience which I had when I thought my offical visit to Puerto Rico was completed and I could return to New York to celebrate Christmas with my wife and our two small boys. It turned out that I could not leave on Christmas Day, but three days later which was the earliest date I could arrange for my arrival home.

Early on that last Sunday morning, the chief of police of the entire island called for me at my hotel and said that we were again going to travel through the central part of the island; but our goal, the chief said, would be explained to me when we arrived at the top of the most prominent section of the island.

Not knowing anything about where we were going, I told the chief and his driver to go right ahead. It was a beautiful day and I was in for what I believed would be a very pleasant trip. However, when we reached what was nearly the last stop, he instructed the driver to park the car. At this point, the chief of police explained why he was taking me on this trip.

Just at that time, I heard sounds from what seemed a church service with the singing of old familiar hymns. I was then told that I had to be exceedingly careful when we were visiting the church and the people who were worshipping there. I was told, "Don't touch anybody. That is, don't shake hands; don't pat children on the head as we usually do. Just sit in the pew and watch the service."

At the close of the morning church program, we were invited to visit this little family—father, mother, and two children—at their home which was just nearby. What a shock it was to me when I realized that I was meeting with not only one family, but a score of families. Adults and little children alike were all afflicted with leprosy. Their faces and their arms and the little children's legs were covered with these huge, ugly-looking growths which, in those days, was practically an incurable disease. After a few minutes of good-byes, I re-entered our automobile and was driven back to San Juan to carry with me for the rest of my life that sad and thoroughly unexpected experience. I learned later that the whole colony of lepers at the top level area of Puerto Rico had been moved by the government to some island in the Pacific Ocean where this and other families similarly affected would spend their entire life known only as "Lepers,"

—Irving T. Gumb
As told to Nan Cooper

NOVEMBER NIGHT

There is a November night that I remember. My father came into my room—very quietly—and helped me dress. Leaving my mother and baby sister asleep, we headed down Main Street. Immediately we could hear the raucous noise of all the factory whistles. Mixed with this jubilation was the cadence of church bells. Our single fire siren played obligato to this throbbing melange of sound. The space around us was charged. Do you know what I mean? Do you remember the fright of ghost stories when you were little? Perhaps not, but this November night held a truly strange, fightening excitement.

Before long, a crowd had gathered where a church and a post office occupied neighboring corners. Here, on a slight rise of ground my dad set me down, with my back against the post office wall. Some of the townspeople had come with lighted torches, causing the mounted police to have difficulty controlling their horses. Alarmed by the smoke and flame, one of the horses whirled away from the crowded intersection, and charged up the bank toward me — ME, — a small five-year-old girl, too frightened to move. Someone whisked me out of the way, but that fear stayed with me for a long time. That night was a celebration of the Armistice signed in November, 1918.

But there was another night, not long after that one, when I learned another kind of fear — fear for a loved one. I woke to the sound of muted voices and a soft light. In the next bed was my baby sister, so sick and weak that she seemed to have stopped breathing. My mother was in the chair beside the bed and our family doctor was sitting on the edge of the bed. Occasionally my mother got a bit of boiled, sweetened water to dribble into the baby's mouth. There was such misery in her eyes when she looked at me that the misery made me afraid.

Much later, I learned that there was nothing more that could have been done for our Ann at that time. During the night the fever broke and the next day she began to recover. But it took a long time, for she had been ill with the "Spanish Influenza."

All over the country, wherever the "doughboys returned home, they carried this virus. It spreads with dismaying speed. The population had no immunity. Sometimes those who cared for the sick were stricken the next day. There was no protection and it could bring death within 24 hours. Families knew the bitter grief of helplessness added to the losses of the war.

These nights I remember are symbols of the joy and sorrow en-

gendered at the signing of the Armistice on November 11, 1918 —
the end of "the war to end all wars" — WW I.

—Janet Norton

V.E. DAY

The day the war ended in the European theatre was May 8, 1945.
I remember it well. I was working in the Alabama Drydocks and
Shipbuilding Company located in Mobile, Alabama. We were
building T-2 tankers for the war effort. This was a big operation
having 25,000 employees working over three shifts. The yard had
four side launching ways and six end launching ways which produced a ship that was 525 feet long and 25,000 tons in weight.
Towards the final months we were producing better than one ship a
month, and finally completed 110 ships before the end of the war
when all further operations were cancelled.

Launch day was an exciting time for everyone. A woman guest
or a sponsor broke the champagne bottle over the bow and called
out, "I christen you 'BEAVER CANYON'" or some other name of
an Indian Battle in our history. The trigger rope was then cut with a
hatchet and the great ship began to move down the greased ways
into the harbor finally pulling free of all cradles and ropes while it
danced on the disturbed waters. Immediately, the big crane lowered
an inner bottom into place for the next ship.

On V.E. Day word came in at midday that the War's end was for
real and the workers laid down their tools and came off the ways,
gathering in front of Way 35. There were cheers, hugs, tears and
great rejoicing. The shipfitters foreman, called "Preacher,"
climbed onto a weldment and let the group in a long prayer of
thanksgiving. Many people got down on their knees in the red dust
of the shipyard as the Preacher gave us his thoughts on this great
day. Many of the workers had husbands, brothers and friends over-
seas and this day meant so much to them.

Slowly the realization that the job is still not complete dawns on
everyone. Japan must be brought to her knees in a long bloody war
and that our tanker program was even more important in the far off

Pacific theatre of war. It was time to go back to work and try harder than ever to make a quality ship in the shortest time possible.

V.E. Day was a very emotional event and it will always be highlighted in my memory. It was while I was working at the Alabama Drydock and Ship Building Company that peace came at the end of World War II.

—Elmer S. Munsell

TEACHING IN THE 1930s

It was a beautiful spring day, sixty years ago. It was an important day. It was the day I was to be interviewed about a teaching position for the fall.

My practice teaching supervisor had arranged an interview for me with the superintendent of schools for an area of Litchfield County in Connecticut where there was a vacancy in Bethlehem Consolidated School. Bethlehem had just consolidated its several one room schools and had built a school with four classrooms. There were to be three teachers in the fall. The fourth room was to be our recreation room on rainy days, and a room for special celebrations or holiday programs.

My class of thirty-three first and second graders arrived in September as excited about going to school as I was about being a teacher.

The children in my classroom were basically in two groups — the ones who lived in the center of town and walked to school and those who lived on the farm just outside of town and walked to school and those who lived on the farms just outside of town, and were transported to school by bus. The children from the farming community spoke little, if any, English. Their parents were Lithuanian and unless there were older brothers and sisters in school this was their first contact with the English language. Remember there were few radios then. Communication was not easy at first but it wasn't long before we were understanding each other and having a great time. They were all eager to learn. I especially enjoyed watching the children helping each other and seeing the shining eyes as speech and word recognition became easier each day. If it seemed that we had reached a stalemate some days, I would go to one of the other class-rooms and recruit some one to translate and intepret for me.

Our school, with the churches and the Grange, was the center for most social activity in the town. We three teachers boarded with a family just down the street from the school and enjoyed planning get-together activities for our combined classes. We also discussed interesting ways to present new material. We were also included in birthday parties and other family celebrations in our pupils' homes. Because we were so close to the community and the families we could better see the needs and problems and help to solve them.

One is drawn to compare education in the 1930's with present day schooling. Today children and teachers have many advantages with beautiful buildings with all kinds of equipment such as projectors, computers, and electronic assistance with tapes, records, art materials, shop equipment, etc.

It appears that the enthusiasm and joy of learning is missing today, except possibly in the lower grades. Children are so far advanced and so sophisticated that such things as Math, Science, Grammar and Geography are boring to them. They are pushed by parents to excel in Athletics, Drama, and a thousand other activites. They have no time to play and grow up naturally.

I enjoyed teaching in Bethlehem, Connecticut for five years. In 1935 Bethehem would not hire a married teacher, so in October I resigned to marry Elmer and move to Norwich, Connecticut.

—Eleanor Munsell

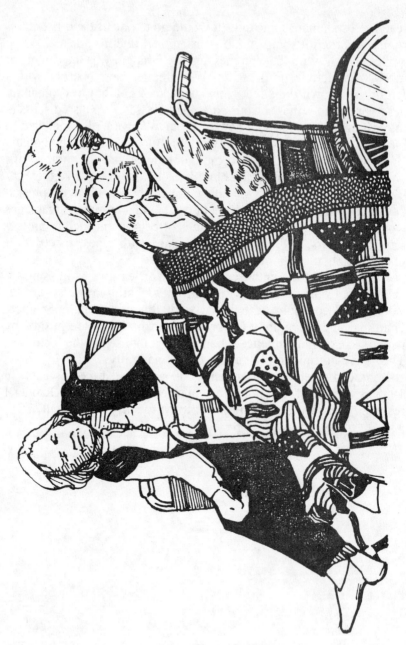

60

Chapter IV

The Pieces of My Life

The stories in this section of the book are really the life experiences that the elderly people remembered. They enjoyed the telling and the students from Marymount redid the stories, working to get additional information to add to the first telling. Some of the storytellers had a stroke that had impaired their speech and they showed the students their life's interests or spoke of them briefly and sometimes haltingly. Students then filled in details, taking the story back to the teller for verification.

A WILDLIFE RETREAT

One summer after my retirement, my time was spent in the forests of the Blue Ridge Mountains of Virginia supervising the building of a second home for my son and his family. This undeveloped parcel of land — some 350 acres — was practically inaccessible, only approachable via winding narrow back roads and then a rock fire trail. I soon learned to dread the roughness of that trail as frequent burst tires became my lot in life.

Our first priority was to bulldoze our way into the site and build an access road, then clear and grade the lot, and get electric lines strung in. Once the A-frame was "under roof" and wired, I moved in a cot and electric grill so I could stay and eliminate the daily 100-mile drive from my home to the building site. That mountain became my home from Memorial Day until Labor Day and I kept busy working with the men on the house, painting, seeding and fertilizing grass, and finally getting a well drilled. The water that well produced was the sweetest and coldest water imaginable.

The A-frame was situated high on the northwest side of the

mountain overlooking the Shenandoah Valley. At night, lights gleaming in the distance enabled us to locate Winchester, Berryville, White Post, and Leesburg, Virginia; Harper's Ferry and Charleston, West Virginia; and a garland of lights marked the course of Interstate 81 up the Valley and Route 50 cutting across the state to West Virginia.

Our mountain retreat soon proved to be a wildlife haven with native animals and birds in abundance sharing the foods provided by nature and our plantings. Birds of every description could be seen: cardinals, blackbirds, doves, scarlet tanagers, orioles, bluebirds, whippoorwills, swallows, phoebes, woodpeckers, many varieties of hawks, owls, and the ever present vultures keeping the forest clean of carrion. Also, the many birds just "passing through" made it a contest to see who could first identify them.

Bobcats raised a pair of kits in their den at the bottom of the clearing; foxes fed their young on chicken scraps left for them on the lawn; and, turkeys shepherded their young through the grain patches planted for their dinners. At night, flying squirrels zoomed onto the tree just off the front deck to eat peanut butter smeared onto the trunk by the grandchildren, while bats performed aerial acrobatics catching insects on the wing. Deer grazed like cattle in the front field (we once counted 23 in the herd) and often bedded down in the grass to sleep several hours before dawn. Possum and groundhog were plentiful, and porcupines, skunks and snakes were something to be avoided.

Black bears occasionally traveled from mountain to mountain in their search for food and would stop to sample the apples on trees planted by some long-gone backwoodsman. On one memorable occasion, a bear ended up staying longer than he anticipated. When I started to enter the garage to get out some equipment, I spotted a hairy black paw sticking out from in front of the tractor. Needless to say, I ventured no closer but "hightailed" it to the other side of the mountain for Pat, a strapping 6-foot-plus neighbor. I'm not exactly "chicken" but I felt reinforcements wouldn't hurt. That hairy foot had not moved in my absence so with great caution we peeked around the tractor. On the floor lay a young black bear which did not respond to careful prodding with a *very long* fishing pole. Our courage restored, we examined the animal and found it had died from a gunshot wound after crawling into the garage to escape its pursuers. A most unfortunate end for this fine animal.

To keep his land at one with nature, my son posts no trespassing signs warning hunters from neighboring forest preserves from shooting game on the property. The animals seem to sense their safety on "our mountain" and it has become our greatest pleasure to sit quietly on the front deck of the A-frame and watch the wildlife going on about their business unafraid and undisturbed.

—H.C. Cregger

A VERY FINE LIFE

My family's from Virginia
Though I was born in Missouri.
In Arlington, I grew up
on a dairy farm, you see.

Old families stick together.
So my husband and I met
as children in the country;
My grandparents knew his grandparents
And our parents too were friends.

That's the way it was in those days.
But I was a happy wife.
He was the very finest man.
I couldn't have asked for a better life.

—Ruth Reeves Lane
As interpreted by Wendy Campbell

SUMMER IN THE COUNTRY

People live quite comfortably in the country, you know. My family comes from Tennessee where I spent most of my early childhood on my Grandmother's farm. I never thought about playmates until I started school. There was just so much to do.

I was allowed to help the men who worked on the farm, and then

I had chores of my own as well. After the chores were done, I would run off to play by myself. We had a very simple life but it was wonderful. I wanted to stay on that farm forever but, when I was six, my mother got after me to go to school.

I still came back to see my Grandmother every summer, though. I would spend the entire summer on the farm. Then, when the harvest was coming in, my mother would call and say that it was time for me to start school.

—Dorothy Karsner
As told to Wendy Campbell

CUPCAKE

Delicate, shell pink
Minature, fragile petals
Lovely creation

—Mark Spies
As interpreted by Kathy Koczyk

About the Author

Mark Spies of Arlington, Virginia has spent the majority of his life involved in engineering. During his college years, he supported himself as a radio DJ at WBL in Decatur, Illinois. Not only did he announce, he also used his knowledge of engineering. After graduation, Mr. Spies accepted a job thirty miles away at another radio station, WDZ. Working again as a DJ, he also built this station's transmitter. In fact, this excellent engineer built his own family's first television set. His qualities were recognized by the Navy when the war occurred. He was subsequently sent to MIT and to Harvard to study radar.

After a full career in the engineering field, Mark Spies retired and immersed himself in roses. He became so interested in roses that he developed his own miniature rose called "Cupcake." The beauty of his rose is depicted in his own Haiku given above.

CHILDHOOD AND CHERRY TREES

I lived in a small town of about 1200 people in Ohio. Everyone knew everything about everybody. One day I took my roller skates and went down a small hill. When I got home, Mother asked me where I had been. She already knew; someone had come by to tell her.

I had a wonderful childhood. I was the oldest of five. There were three girls first and we finally had a boy and then another boy to carry on the Dietrich name. You'd have thought that heaven had broken loose, my father was so excited. We lived in a big Victorian house with a parlor for special occasions and a porch on the corner of the house. We could see all the way to Five Corners from the yard. The streets joined together and the lots were shaped so that our backyard backed up to our grandparents' and we could smell the good smells when my grandmother was cooking. She was a wonderful cook and we could always stop in when we knew that she was cooking.

We had 22 cats and finally my mother said that we couldn't have any more. One day I was standing in some tall grass and a little kitten came bounding throught the grass toward me and followed me home. When I got home, my mother said, "Marie, I have told you, no more cats," but I said that the cat came to me. She let me keep just this one more.

My mother did her best to make a lady out of me. She taught me to play the organ. We had an old-fasioned pump organ and I could barely reach the pump pedals. In spite of all her efforts, I was always where I wasn't supposed to be. My mother called me "Tommie" because I was such a tomboy. Mother had three girls and two boys but I was her tomboy. The second daughter was a real lady, but the third was a tomboy, too, and I used to take her to climb up telephone poles (remember when they had spikes on them?). She was afraid that we'd fall, but it never even occurred to me and we never did, though we had to reach way up from one spike to another. That sister was about four years younger than I, so I guess she could have fallen. Down below our yard there were hillocks, and we'd jump from one to another and sometimes we'd land in swampy water. We'd come home dirty as could be, but Mother was young and enjoyed fun herself. I don't remember her ever spanking us. My father made his own ice cream and shipped it all over Ohio. It was good. He made some with egg whites, but never gave anyone the recipe. Our home was a happy one.

—Marie Detrick Sprigg
As told to Jan Vincent

AFGHANS

I never walked my afghans
I never fed them, too
In fact I never talked to them
Even though some were blue!

The truth is some were white and
brown with a yellowish-greenish hue.
The one hundred and fifty that weakened
my hands are now covering some of you!

Squaring Granny was very tough,
But not as hard as rippling.
Crocheting gave in to needlepoint
Which thankfully is not crippling.

I still have three of my afghans
Though needlepoint is my feat.
So while one may warmly cover you
The other may serve as your seat!!

—Ruth Fitzmorris
As adapted by Kathy Koczyk

SHIPYARD DAYS

In the early stages of organizing the shipyards at the beginning of World War II, it became apparent that man power would be a major problem. After the physical plant was built which involved the construction of six end launching ways along with twelve gantry steam cranes, outfitting docks and a dry dock large enough to handle ships of large sizes were also required. Various buldings for fabrication, a mold loft and administrative offices were also needed. Fortunately, many of these items were available at the old Alabama Shipbuilding operations.

Widespread recruiting was only partially successful and a program was started to hire blacks and train them to handle tradesman jobs such as welding, ship fitting, chippers and grinders. When the first of these men were put to work, a nasty race riot resulted and at this point, the government called two of the largest construction companies on the east coast and arranged to make them joint partners with Alabama Drydock. The partners concluded that the four site launching ways in the North Yard would become exclusively black workmen with white foremen to supply the skills necessary for the training that would be required. This arrangement proved to be successful for the most part during the rest of the operation. The first ship launched in the North Yard took almost a year to pass inspection.

This situation was corrected shortly, however, when the same men launched a ship in twenty-eight days which was the same time as the White yard. Black workers became excellent skilled welders. They seemed to pick up the skill with speed and soon became fine workers in the shipbuilding process.

Every person hired for welding or tacking jobs was put through an intensive training course in special booths to practice welding in all the positions. This included engineers and administrators who were given an intensive orientation in welding, as well as, all phases of the work in the ship yard. This allowed a construction supervisor to acquire the ability to plan and lead the various operations under the eyes of the old hands at shipbuilding. We learned fast despite some burns on our pants and some eye irritation from welding flash. Soon we were calling the wall a bulkhead, and vertical plates in the inner bottoms became floors, while floors became decks.

One interesting operation in shipbuilding was called "shake down cruise." This was a testing procedure where every aspect of the ship's operation was given a test under the severest conditions. One test was called the "hog and sag" in which an attempt to break the ship in half was made by pumping the forward and aft tanks full of water and leaving center tanks empty. The reverse effect was also made by emptying the fore and aft tanks and by filling the center tanks. This test was considered so severe that the ship was placed in drydock and every seam was looked over for any defects in welding that the test might have caused.

Another test was called the "crash test." Here the ship was placed on a straight course full ahead. It was then sent into reverse at full power. The result was extreme vibration throughout the ship and would bring out any imperfections in the work. All the machinery for the ship was tested including navigational equipment and all the guns were tested and fired. Logs were kept of all gauges and thermometers.

The test that I was involved in went on all night and took us deep into the Gulf of Mexico. We had a harbor pilot on the bridge and a Norwegian gun crew manning our armament as well as a Norwegian captain. This crew was present because there were plans to turn the ship over to the Norwegian government for use in the battles of the Atlantic. Every young engineer loved to go on these "shake down cruises" because of the excitement and the chance to learn.

—Elmer S. Munsell

A WONDERFUL LIFE

I have had a wonderful life. I was born on March 15, 1892, in Jackson, Mississippi. It was the "Ides of March." My father was so proud of Jackson, which was a small town. He was the clerk of the court there.

I went to a little country school, the boys could throw balls over the roof of it. I guess I learned the ABC's and how to write.

I remember blocks of ice were being used to keep things cold. They were brought to the house in the ice wagon, in a box covered in sawdust. The men would move the boxes and put them down.

I remember when people quilted quilts. The girls would get together to make them for people who needed them. We had hope chests, but I don't remember what we put in them.

I met my husband in Jackson. He was a wonderful person. He went to Washington to see about joining the Army in the War to

End All Wars, but the Navy needed him. He was a chaplain in the Navy, and went all around the world. We had children but I followed him around as much as I could. He always teased me and would say, "You are twelve days older than I." I guess that meant I was supposed to be wiser or something.

—Ellen Thomas

COON HUNTING

I lived with my grandmother from the age of eight or nine until it was time to go to college. I helped Uncle Simon with the farm work, which included raising crops such as wheat, oats, buckwheat, corn, potatoes, and cabbage. The grains would go to the grist mill to be ground into flour and into corn meal used for making cornbread. The cabbages would be made into kraut at the local factory. Much hard work went into running a farm and you had to make your own fun.

During my teens, my favorite "fun" was coon hunting at night with Uncle Simon in the dense woods covering the hills near my grandmother's house. We did not really hunt the coons, as we did not take any guns with us, but we used coonhounds to track the coons. Our chase was made by four black-and-tan Redbone hounds whose "tongueing" (barking) could be heard for miles while they trailed the scent of the coons. The coon would eventually tire of the game and climb a tree to evade the hounds. In the tree, the coon's black masked face could be seen peering through the leaves as it rested on the branch of the tree.

Our tracking often lasted from nine or ten until nearly dawn. Many a night, I would curl up on a pile of leaves and nap while waiting for the hounds to chase the coon back around to us.

Occasionally we would capture a young coon. We would cage the captured coon and make it into a pet. Our coon hunts were fun; also, they provided good exercise for the hounds.

—Hugh Creeger

TRAVEL

Around the world
So new, so safe
Meeting people
In every place

Planes offered coupons
To keep whistles wet
I gave mine to others
While I just set

Working for public health
I traveled alone
But not for long
Since the world is my home

— *Marie Dougherty*
As adapted by Kathy Koczyk

MY STORY

I grew up in Ohio but even as a child I longed to travel. I had an aunt who lived in Annandale, Virginia and my mother gave me permission to come to Virginia. I wanted to be a nurse but my mother was set against this and felt that studying at the Washington School for Secretaries would introduce the business world to me.

During the week, I would live with my cousins downtown and on the weekend, I would go out to Annandale with Aunt Pearl. On Saturdays, a friend and I would go down to Haines Point to ride horses. One Saturday, we encountered burning trash on the bridle path. My horse suddenly stopped, but I did not. I was not badly hurt when I landed and so with reins in hand, I walked back to the stables near the Lincoln Memorial.

My Aunt Pearl introduced me to the man who lived across the road from her. We later married but he turned out to be the wrong man for me. He left and I had to make my own way.

Since I could not be a nurse, I did the next best thing. I went to work at the Visiting Nurses Association. I was very successful in

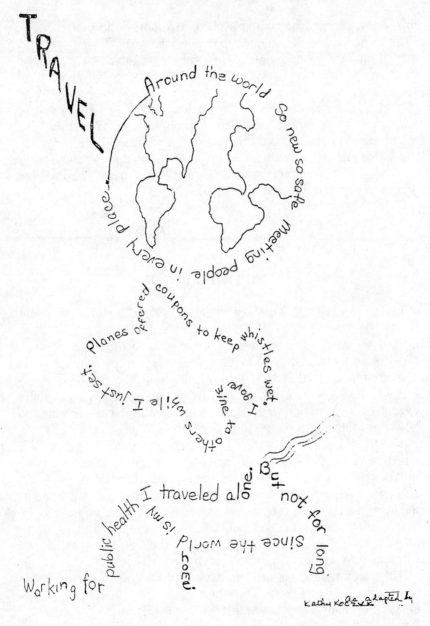

TRAVEL

Around the world so new so safe

Meeting people in every place.

Planes offered coupons to keep whistles wet.
I gave to others while I just set.

But not for long. Since the world is my home. I traveled alone.

Working for public health

Kathy Koren adapted by

this work, going from being a clerk to running the entire office. With a friend, I took a major trip every other year. Twice, we traveled around the world by plane. In Taiwan, we took a strenuous trip by train. At this time, travel of this sort was somewhat unusual for single women.

When I returned each time, there were many groups of people who came to see my slides. The Ashton Heights Women's Club asked me to conduct programs showing my slides. To this day, all the slides are numbered with descriptions written for each slide.

Now, I live at the Powhatan Center with many friends with whom I can share my stories.

—*Marie Sprigg*
As told to Kathy Koczyk

LITTLE DID I KNOW

I was born in 1892. One day when I was ten years old, my father made a wooden box, oh, about three feet wide. He instructed me as to how to make rope handles on either side of the box. He said, "We're going to let you go to a boys summer camp *all by yourself*. The camp is located in New Hampshire on the shores of Winnepasacke." In the year I am talking about almost no one was there except for occasional visits from Indians. Why I was chosen and how I got there from home in Massachusetts I shall never know.

The year was 1902. At the age of ten, I was young for camp life which was usually organized for boys of twelve years. We were instructed in the art of setting up tents. I soon learned that I would be there for ten weeks. I was unknown to other youngsters and to the men in charge. For ten weeks I would be sleeping on the ground with a little rubber blanket beneath me. I was told not to worry about the wind and the rain because they picked a spot that sloped from head to foot gradually so that the rain would run off.

Then they taught me my first lesson in how to camp out in the open with no protection. They taught me how to make a "*hip-hole.*" For many years I used that bit of information to good results. After you decided exactly how you were going to lie down, the hip-hole was located exactly where one your of hips would be. You

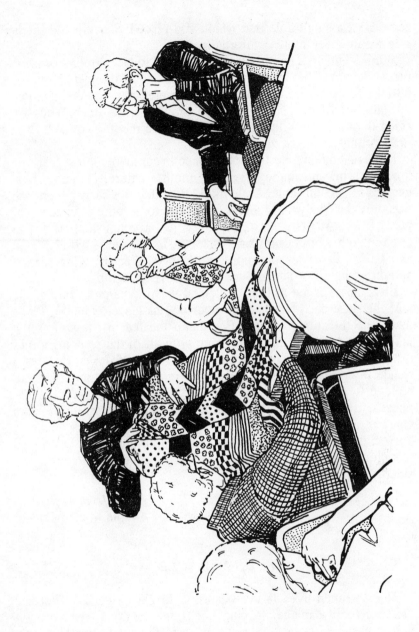

carved out a small hole into which you placed your hip and therefore would sleep more comfortably.

But I was taught another lesson for I had to sleep in that position for ten weeks. That lesson was to follow one of the instructors out into the forest where a lot of pine trees were growing. We gathered up handfuls of pine needles which grow on pine trees. Thus we filled the hip-hole with pine needles to give it some comfort for a tired youngster of ten years to flop into bed.

I was just having my first experience in eating outdoors, learning how to swim and many lessons of mother nature, including pine needles for the hip-hole. Little did I know that this early experience was only the first year of a series that was to become a sixteen-year way of life. At first, of course, I was just a youngster selected to live with other boys of my own age; but, in due time I worked as an assistant to the older and more experienced men in taking care of and directing all of the activities for the whole camp.

I was an assistant at first but later I was in charge of one of the tents because each tent had an older boy as leader. Finally, I was made the director of a very fine camp located in Massachusetts; and, I was directing that boys camp with all of the responsibilities of taking care of the usual contingent of 150 boys. It was this experience in boys camp that finally gave me the opportunity to enter college — Brown University — and it helped to pay *all* my expenses — this meant tuition, clothing, books, dormitory room charges, and food. So I have always loved the outdoor life and have appreciated what I learned there. The opportunity that developed from it and the college education I received have benefited me ever since.

— Irving T. Gumb
As told to Nan Cooper

FOUR MIRACLES

Three women lived in this beautiful, bright room. The first had suffered brain damage, leaving her sound of mind, but with severely impaired speech. She was able to formulate thoughts only with great difficulty and very slowly. The second was immobilized by a creeping paralysis that had not quite reached her warm smile or the gracious movement of her head. The third lay in a catatonic trance, a small motionless figure in a bed made enormous by her tininess.

The music began, and at the first sounds of the zither, the first lady sighed as a wave of relaxation passed over her strained features. The paralyzed lady began to hum, then to sing and make requests. Despite the stiffening lungs, her voice changed miraculously from soft and husky to full and clear. It was a lovely thing to hear her sing.

Then, another miracle happened when the first lady suddenly sang a folksong through all the verses, clearly and with expression. She requested more songs and sang them easily and confidently. Nurses gathered spellbound in the doorway; they could not believe their ears were hearing correctly.

As the music continued, sounds that seemed to come from the catatonic lady announced the beginning of the third miracle. Incredibly, the sounds *were* coming from her—inarticulate, but unmistakably related to the music, in a pattern exactly matching the rhythm of each song or piece. Suddenly she sat bolt upright, eyes wide open, and nurses rushed in to elevate the bed behind her back. She sat up, she participated, for the further hour or so that the music continued. At the last, when the zither was put away and the musician was departing, she looked up eye-to-eye, meaningfully, making sounds with the exact cadence of "thank you very much."

And what was the fourth miracle? That miracle happened within the musician. Not only well-known and often played music, but long forgotten pieces, songs heard but never before played came to the player. Unprepared music with difficult harmonizations; all came in a rich stream, entered mind and fingers and flowed out in the zither's haunting chiaroscuro in the most perfect form, without any conscious effort.

I believe in the four miracles, because I am the musician who played that day. In my memory there will always be four women in that beautiful room, and four miracles.

—Jane Curtis

AN UNEXPECTED TRIP

It was a beautiful day, sunshine and blue skies. I was about eight years old; and one of my cousins was 11 or so. My Uncle Otto and two other cousins were with us and there had been great excitement as we planned this trip.

We had left home at eight o'clock in the morning, hoping to go sight seeing in Washington for the day. Sometime during our morning excursion, someone came up to us to give us tickets for a trip down the river on the old Charlie Werner, the boat at the dockside. We took them of course, and once aboard, we settled down for a fine ride in the spring sunshine. There were many people aboard and everyone was laughing and enjoying themselves.

Toward early afternoon the sun darkened. Slowly, it became very dark, and the wind began coming from the Northwest part of the city. It began to rain. Suddenly, the wind blew hard and the sky grew threateningly dark.

All the people on board hurried into the ship's chambers. Then, to our amazement, we heard a loud noise as though something had burst. Everyone knew that there was equipment down below, and we realized that the boiler had probably burst. There was steam rising into the air as the engines began to gasp their last breath. Men traveling alone, jumped up leaving women and children to fend for themselves. All were praying that they would make it to shore.

However, we soon became stuck on the shore of the river where the captain, in his wisdom, had steered the boat for its safety. We stayed there for about three hours, before a Coast Guard boat rolled up with the intention of pulling the Charlie Werner out of the river.

People were getting very hungry and were quite uneasy about being rescued by the Coast Guard cutter. Finally, the Coast Guard crew put boards from the Cutter to the ship in which we were marooned. Everyone waited anxiously for help; and all were finally boarded on the Coast Guard ship and taken to the shore leading to the hotel. People walked on the plank from the ship to the shore and my cousin and I were led to the plank first. All women and children were first taken off the ship and carried to the shore, where we stayed waiting for the men to get off too.

The men got off the ship and tried to get a boat to go across the river to the Army reservation on the other side. It was very dark and, the sky was clouded and looked VERY, VERY ominous, to say the least. However, finding a boat was more difficult than they had expected. Finally, the men succeeded in locating a dingy. They got into the small craft and began to row across the dark and menacing Potamac River to the Army installation. It was a frightening situation for all concerned.

The men in the dingy reached the other side of the river. One of them went searching for a larger craft that would hold the passengers awaiting rescue on the other side of the river. A large boat was located and the men were able to come back to the hotel sooner then we had expected.

Back at the hotel on shore, the hotel manager, Mr. Schabe had been able to secure food for the group of people who waited for the return of the men from across the river. This created much better feelings among the holiday group.

ALL ABOARD! Traveling the dark, dark river, we finally reached the Army installation. We walked in heavy mud and, with weary footsteps, for about half a mile to the electric railroad that would take us to Washington. Eventually, we arrived safe and sound at home but everyone was very tired.

The store on the corner was still open because they had a telephone ready to receive any message that might come from the travelers. The store owner, Mr. Sam Bondarff, kept the store open because there was a telephone there for information in case anyone heard from the missing passengers. How happy we were to see our mothers and our families. We were pretty much disheveled and our mothers were distraught from waiting so long to hear from their loved ones. It was surely a trip to remember.

—Erna G. Garner

Chapter V

Imported Quilt Pieces

Several stories and poems that have been developed by persons in the very old category have been made available to the author. These people were not members of the Powhatan Nursing Group, but fall well within the 86 year old average of the group. These individuals wrote because they wished to share an experience in some form with the younger generation. Hopefully, you will enjoy these pieces also.

MY MEMORY OF MEMORIAL DAY

I have been wondering lately what has happened to Memorial Day. It is still a national holiday, but doesn't seem to mean much any more, especially to the younger generation. And, it ought to mean more and more as the years go by. But it seems as though it is just a day to be free from school for the children, and I expect there are many parents who would be glad if it weren't so. When I was a youngster, it seems as though our elders worked at making the day mean something to us.

During the most of my school days we lived in Westport, and the day was made much of there. (I wonder if it still is.) Of course, the day was a holiday, there was no school as such, but we were off to school at just about the regular time just the same. One great difference being that that morning we were dressed in out best, and many of our parents went with us to hear the program of patriotic songs and "pieces" for which we had been preparing for several weeks. I remember one year I "spoke" the poem, "Hats Off" and I still remember the first verse, which is:

"Hats Off!
Along the street there comes
The blare of bugles, the ruffle of drums,
A flash of color beneath the sky,
Hats Off! The flag is passing by."

And my sister Fleda, one year, gave the poem, "Barbara Fritchie". The school auditorium which was the large high school room, was always well filled and at the close of the program, we all lined up for the big event of the day—that was the parade to the cemetery.

Civil War veterans and later the Spanish American War veterans were there in uniform, and as I remember it, it seems as though just about every veteran in the community must have been present. One veteran led the parade, proudly carrying the large flag; and how my childish heart swelled as I saw its beautiful colors rippling in the breeze. The band followed close behind the flag-bearer. The old soldiers in their blue uniforms followed, and I remember yet how we almost reverenced anyone wearing our country's uniform. Then came the school children, and how we all loved to step off in time to the beat of the drum. I don't remember in what order as to age or sex we marched, but most of us were there. (We wouldn't have missed it for anything.) I think Westport must have been proud of its school children in those days, for we were all dressed in our best clothes, AND behavior. I don't remember what the boys best clothes looked like, but about the same as today, I suppose. The girls were mostly dressed in white, starched, and often ruffled, summer dresses. Just about every child had a bouquet of flowers of some sort, with lilacs usually predominant. A few of the soldiers carried several small flags.

When we arrived at a central spot in the cemetery, the parade stopped, and after a prayer and a brief speech on patriotism, we fanned out and laid flowers on as many graves as we could. The veterans put the new flags on the graves of all the soldiers buried there, and removed the old ones. There was an orderliness, a quietness, and solemnity to the whole proceeding that somehow helped us to realize a little more what sacrifices had been made for our country, and for us. In that way, Memorial Day was more than just a day on which we didn't have to go to school. It had a special significance for us. After the flowers and flags had been distributed, we all left the cemetery quietly and went our various ways for the rest of the day.

—Helen Moss

75 YEARS OF THE WASHINGTON PARADE

I was only about four years old at Taft's inauguration, but I remember father commenting on Taft's misfortune with the weather for his parade. Several years later, I remember watching as Mr. Hostetler, the father of a good friend, set up the ladies for another parade. He was quite an activist. I remember him walking through the crowd of women and handing each a banner. In the end they gave him one and, on March 3, 1916, the Suffragettes marched for women's rights with Mr. Hostetler in their midst, holding high a banner proclaiming, "MEN CAN VOTE. WHY CAN'T I?"

I was at Arlington Cemetery for the burial of the Unknown Soldier following WWI. One of my friends told me years later that foreign newsmen had been puzzled by the headlines the day after the event but I had understood. They read, "OYSTER BARS JAM PROBE!" You see, there was a D.C. commissioner named Oyster who had stopped the investigations into the incredible traffic jams surrounding Arlington Cemetery that day. Father was bringing an elderly neighbor, but he let mother, me, and my sister off at the 14th Street bridge and we walked across the fields to the cemetery. We weren't the only ones either, I can tell you. I recognized some of the justices of the Supreme Court as I crossed the field. They had had to walk too. It was worth it though. I'll never forget that moment, looking out over the city of Washington while they played taps.

Mother hapened to be interested in politics. I was going to Central High School in 1918-1920 when mother got into going down to the Senate Gallery. My sister and I would meet her there after our last call. We got quite good at watching for people leaving so we could get better and better seats. By the end of many afternoons, we would be right down in front. That is how it came about that I was in the Senate Gallery when the League of Nations was presented on the floor. What a spectacle! The entire gallery rose and cheered when Senator Lodge and Sentor Borah spoke. When Senator Hitchcock spoke, the galleries hissed. Nowadays we'd say that there were activists in the galleries, but it's not true. It was a spontaneous demonstration of feeling from the spectators. That kind of thing rarely makes it into the history books.

Washington was an interesting place to grow up. I lived on Irving Street in Mount Pleasant as a girl. I can remember, mornings, watching Senator Borah of Idaho ambling down Irving Street on his horse which he kept stabled nearby.

Although my family moved to Chicago, I returned to D.C. after completing four years of work at Stanford University. I lived at Stoneleigh Court, not far from the Mayflower Hotel. It was 1942. I just had a room, no cooking privileges, so I had to eat out. Sunday I'd walk out to the Mayflower, get my Sunday Post, and go in for a good breakfast. There was a gentleman always there before me. He sat in the same place every Sunday. It was the waitress who pointed out that, in that seat, he could only be approached from the front. It was J. Edgar Hoover

I began working for the government during the war. I remember one rather fun incident very clearly. Mrs. Roosevelt was going to receive the "Women of the Government" at an afternoon reception. One of my friends commented that "Oh, (she'd) so love to go and be received by Mrs. Roosevelt." My office had been given several tickets and by a trickle down effect, my friend received one on the day of the event. She refused to go! She felt that she "hadn't dressed for the White House" so she gave the ticket to me. Well, I felt that Mrs. Roosevelt and the other ladies wouldn't care a hoot what Janet Murray was wearing so off I went. A nice young Marine took us up one by one to meet Mrs. Roosevelt and the ladies of the Cabinet. We all said, "How do you do" to each other all the way down the line. "How-de-do, How-de-do, How-de-do, howdedo, howdedo . . ." It sounded like the seashore.

Living where I do now, across from the Capitol Hilton, it's easy for me to get places and keep in touch with things as they happen. I could look out my window to see what Lady Bird Johnson's inaugural ball gown was like (and then go later to the Smithsonian and see it up close). I remember when Nixon stayed at the Capitol Hilton. We were all lined up behind ropes in the lobby to see him. He went down the entire line with his hand outstretched, but no one reached to shake it.

I have seen all of the inaugural parades in recent years. I listen to the TV and then I know just when to go down to Pennsylvania Avenue to see the newly inaugurated President pass by. Did I tell you how cross I was at the Carters? I had my little pattern. When they left the Capitol, I'd go down to see the parade. But the Carters walked, you see, and I could only see the tops of their heads!

The last time with the Reagans, I wasn't so concerned with seeing the President, but I did want to see his horses. So, I went on down beyond the White House, and, while the President was in his reviewing stand, I got beautiful views of those lovely horses.

—Janet Murray

MOVING OUT OF SIGHT

A shrouded world my eyes survey
And that at best is thru a haze
How hard my brain must strain to weigh
The clouded, bent, enfeebled rays.

Dark shadows settle on the stage
Where actors and faces blend
Bold print gets blurred upon the page
On tape recordings I depend

I scan the food upon my plate
No recognition in my gaze
Sight, taste and smell must all debate
What seems most like a bouillabaisse

In conquering the bleak subway
I clutch the rail or hug the wall

And when steep stairs come into play
Cane takes me down to spare a fall

As planetary view recedes
My cosmic sphere approaches nigh
Suffice the memory of hold deeds
They tempt no longer failing eyes.

—Edward Gottlieb

OUR TEACHER

As measured by the television range
Her life by work or step is quite confined
Yet in her hands she holds the strings of change
That guide your hearts through realms of humankind

She prods young minds beyond the conscious ledge
Inspiring each to shun the passive role
Then intellect transcending drives a wedge
So conscience be the lever of the soul

So much her bold exploring mind exacts
She grants the casual but off-stage parts
Begrudging every tick that time subtracts
As seeds of growth propel adventurous hearts
Her classroom has a skylight to the world
And on her blackboards dreams of men unfurled

—Edward Gottlieb

FAREWELL VIA PUBLIC ADDRESS SYSTEM

I'll miss your hurry down the street
And bright "Good Morning" at the door,
Your stairway tramp of merry feet, —
These cheerful sounds I'll hear no more.

Will you recall the P.A. voice
The plea to sit up straight and tall;

Each message that should guide your choice
To climb new heights, to heed a call?

I'll think of you with book-bag full
Your white shirts on assembly day,
With fondness for each tug and pull
That brought us close in secret play.

Remember How I shared your top or ball,
Rejoiced to hear you laugh and sing;
Remember how I hushed you in the hall,
To every joyous memory cling!

—Edward Gottlieb

Note: Used with permission from American Educator.

Normally, *American Educator* does not print poetry. We've made an exception for Edward Gottlieb. As a New York City school teacher, he first joined the teacher union movement in 1926 as a member of the New York Teachers Union, an early forerunner of the United Federation of Teachers/AFT. In 1960, as a school principal at P.S. 165 during the first New York City teachers strike, he joined the picket line and was one of a handful of principals who resisted board of education demands that the names of striking teachers be turned over to the board. At a time when many other principals punished teachers they knew to be union members with poor class assignments and additional duties, Gottlieb always encouraged teachers at his school to join the then small uynion. Just as importantly—and just as unpopularly—he encouraged teachers to pursue innovations to improve education. As one teacher who worked with him said, "There was a feeling of freedom and latitude in the schools; we did not feel hidebound to follow certain ways."

Mr. Gottlieb is now retired, in his eighties, and going blind. Always a Renaissance man, he is still a poet.

Reprinted, with permission, from the Spring 1988 issue of AMERICAN EDUCATOR, the quarterly journal of the American Federation of Teachers.

ADVENTURES IN A CASTLE IN SPAIN

I can't say I've been deprived when it comes to travel. I've been many places in my life and had many adventures. One time, I remember, I was locked away in a castle in Spain: It happened this way:

I was traveling in Spain on my own, quite a few years back now, when I reached an old fortress, high on a hill. It was called the Fortress of Coruna and was separated from the little town of Coruna by a long walkway. I decided to walk up and see what it was like. There was a guard at the doorway but he let me in. I asked him what time they closed up for the night and was told that they would be closing at 4:30. I was quite pleased as that gave me several hours to wander at my leisure. I had a wonderful time especially out on the ramparts of the fortress. At about 4:15 I returned to the great hall, where, to my dismay, I discovered the massive gates to the fortress locked and barred. I had been closed in!

WELL! I considered my plight for a few minutes. Even if I yelled no one would hear me through the massive doors or stone walls and over that long causeway. However, I had benches to sleep on and I knew that there were "facilities". Things could have been worse. As I prepared to spend a long, cold, hungry night in my Spanish fortress, I looked again at the massive door. Although I'm a small person, I decided that I might just be able to move the large wooden bars holding the doors shut. With some effort, and after a little time, I was successful. As I stepped out onto the causeway and into the Spanish twilight, I didn't consider the fact that I now was in no position to lock the doors again. I pushed them shut, of course, but when I was halfway down the causeway I looked back and saw the great gates of the Fortress swinging wide open. I've always wondered what the authorities made of that the next day.

—Janet Murray

DISCIPLINE, THE OLD FASHIONED WAY

Springtime is here again, and as always it brings maple-sugaring time to the North Country. And, thoughts of maple sugar just about always bring to my mind the first time I ever remember tasting that delicacy.

It was way back in 1898 and I should imagine just about this time of year. We lived in the town of Lewis, in a neighborhood known as "Stowersville". I had started to school the September before when I was still five, (I was six in February). It was the second year of school for my sister, Fleda (now Mrs. Charles Cleland of Lewis), who was one and one-half years older than I. We carried our lunches to school, and on this day which I remember so well, my mother had given us each an apple, for which apparently there was no room in our pails.

When recess time came I took my apple from my desk, and was rubbing it and looking at it, enjoying it in anticipation, and perhaps deciding where to take the first bite, when Fleda grabbed the apple and said it was hers. Of course, I denied it — insisted it was mine — that I had taken it from my desk where it had been all morning, but she insisted it was hers — that it must be because she couldn't find hers anywhere. And, though I cried and made quite a fuss, she kept the apple and ate it all, not giving me even one bite. (It must be that the teacher decided to let us fight it out, for I don't remember her doing anything about it).

Noon came and Fleda finished eating her lunch first, and started to bundle up to go out to play, and when she put on her coat she discovered an apple in the pocket. Of course she was surprised, and though I insisted she should give it to me in place of mine which she had eaten, she refused saying, "No, you can't have it. THIS apple is MINE, for I remember now I put my apple in my pocket." And in spite of my tears and cries and scoldings (and I guess there was quite a fuss made by one six-year old) she ate all the apple, and again refused me even a bite. Apparently the teacher still didn't interfere to settle the argument, but she evidently did feel sorry for me, for she told me, "Not to mind", and she gave me a sandwich from her lunch pail.

That sandwich! I'll never forget it! It was made from home-made bread (no store bread then), a thick-spreading of home-made butter (no margarine), and a generous layer of soft maple sugar. Good? I think I had never eaten anything that tasted quite so good. If I had, the taste of that sandwich was so different from anything I had ever had that the delicious, delicate sweetness of it still lingers in my mind; and, for years everything I ate suffered in comparison with the flavor of that sandwich.

—Helen Moss

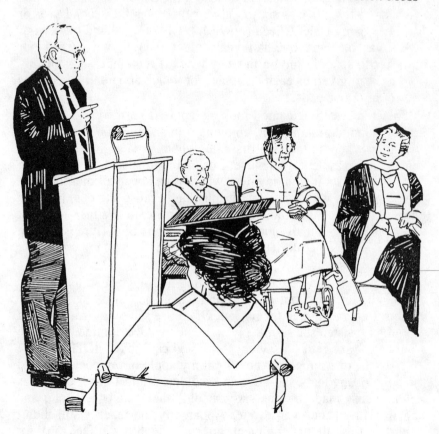

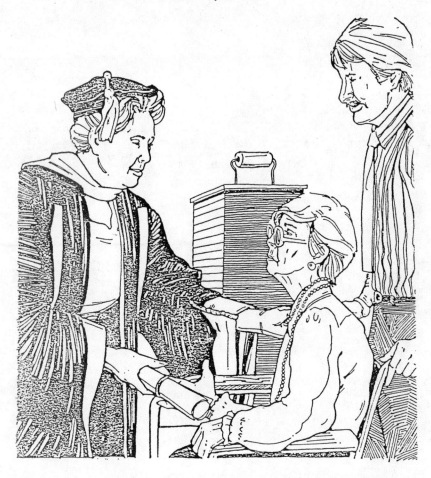

Chapter VI

Making the Border of the Quilt

You have read the stories that the elderly folks at Powhatan Nursing home produced with the assistance of the Marymount University graduate students. There are several features of these stories that are worth an additional comment. The stories are nearly all positive ones. It is not that these very old individuals have not experienced difficulties. Indeed, some of them were telling their stories from wheelbeds or wheelchairs. Several had suffered from strokes and others were somewhat physically incapacitated, but they did not focus on these recent difficulties. The predominant theme was that they had had a good life and had enjoyed the passage of it. Perhaps there is a lesson in this for all of us.

A second idea comes through in these stories. It is that the really worthwhile things are remembered and worth telling about. This group of people has lived through several wars, including World War I and World War II; the Great Depression, and an enormous number of technological changes. The only stories dealing with war are those where some personal, satisfactory experience was remembered. The direct relationship to war and the tragedy of it were not the focus of the stories.

In the *Bible*, there are several references to the fact that there are unchanging verities. In the Book of Hebrews, for example, there is a reference in Ch. 12:26-27 to those things which can be shaken (created things) — "so that those which cannot be shaken may remain." The stories overall are about unchanging, unshakeable relationships, such as family, good times with friends, favorite pastimes and the experiences from which they have learned much. Perhaps during the last few years, the shakeable, created things have become ordered at a lower level and the elderly person sees with a sixth sense that which really matters. They have lived many years and the years teach. This group of people understands the real values and now in the later years of life, they focus on these changeless values. Perhaps this is the stage of life where there is actually a higher level of cognitive development. At this stage the individual focuses on simplification, not simple ideas but rather, "on the things in life that are more meaningful to the person" (John, 1988, p. 30).

It might be worth noting also, that the vocabulary and the grammar in the stories are of good quality. It belies the conception that elderly people are no longer able to function intellectually. The ideas flow together well and there are places in the stories where humor as well as happiness can be seen.

CONTINUE THE WORK

The procedures used in getting the stories for this book can be used by any group of people who are interested in the history of their immediate area or of a particular group. Students from high schools, or colleges, could collect the stories from people in the nursing homes in their area. Girl Scout groups could seek out elders in the community and learn from them as they listen to the stories the older people tell. Church groups or synagogue members could gather information about their congregations, and a history of such groups would be of interest to the present members.

If you have an older relative who has an excellent memory, why not record the stories that this person can tell? In the years to come, this can serve as anecdotal history. Sometimes, there are bits of information about the family that are held by one particular family member. In my family, we always ask Aunt Goldie about things like "who is related to whom." These pieces of information need to be recorded for use over the years.

Write the stories, and in the writing, enjoy the flavor of days gone by; sense the love of family and friends; and think long about the stories you will tell when you are older yourself.

BIOGRAPHICAL SKETCHES

The elderly people involved in this process:

Elizabeth Ellen Sullivan Coulon was born in Washington, D.C. in 1906. She has raised a son and a daughter, lived through two world wars and is an active participant in our weekly class discussions. Her poem, *The Age of Invention,* clearly reflects her facility with words.

Hugh C. Cregger was a delightful individual born in 1903. A prolific writer, he kept his fellow residents amused and thrilled with his tales of adventure and intriguing life stories. We are lucky enough to have two of Mr. Cregger's efforts included in this book.

Jane Curtis was born in Illinois but she earned a BA from Wellesley College in Massachusetts. Later an MA and a PhD from the Catholic University were added to her educational background. She's worked as a musician, translator and analyst and has volunteered her time working in the longterm care field as a nursing home advocate unter Northern Virginia Longterm Care Ombuds program and under Loudoun County Area Agency on Aging.

Marie Doughety was born in Pennsylvania on February 1, 1897. She worked as a government nurse, and as she puts it, "During WWI, I was too busy to have a hobby." Marie was a world traveler, loving life and people everywhere.

Ruth Fitzmorris was born in New York On August 14, 1914. She moved to Arlington, VA as a new bride. Although caring for her home was a full time job, she managed time to develop an interest in crocheting, needlepoint, and ceramics.

Erna Garner was born in Washington, D.C. in May of 1904. She worked as a legal stenographer and law researcher in the Department of Justice for 20 years. Thereafter, she was self-employed, working for a lawyer for many years. From 1930 to 1957 she was principal soprano soloist in large churches in the area, and retired in 1988 after singing at senior citizen groups. As Erna puts it, "I've had a good life!"

Edward Gottlieb was a New York City school teacher. He first joined the teacher union movement in 1926 as a member of the New York Teachers Union, an early forerunner of the United Federation of Teachers/AFT. In 1960, as a school principal at P.S. 165 during the first New York City teachers' strike, he joined the picket line and was one of a handful of principals who resisted board of education demands that the names of striking teachers be turned over to the board. As one teacher who worked with him said, "There was a feeling of freedom and latitude in the schools; we did not feel hidebound to follow certain ways." Always a Renaissance man, he is still a poet.

Irving T. Gumb, born in 1892, is now, and always has been, one of the world's priceless individuals. At the end of a very long and exciting life, he retains a supremely active mind, though nearly blind. Mr. Gumb was recently asked to officiate at ceremonies for the 1987-88 graduating class at Marymount University, an undertaking at which he excelled. We are proud to present two of Mr. Gumb's short stories.

Dorothy Karsner is a bright and twinkling individual. Born in 1910, she raised two children with the wonderful Kentucky boy she tells of meeting in a Washington, D.C. hostelry. The two stories submitted by Mrs. Karsner reflect both country and city joys, and show that even the simplest reflections can be wonderfully interesting.

Elsie Marvin has wonderful memories of her youth in California. Her stories about her family, always told with a twinkle and a smile, are wonderfully graphic. *The Dance of a Lifetime* reflects several of her tales.

Helen Moss was born in 1892 and lived in the Adirondack Mountains most of her life. She was a farmer's wife and after her husband's death maintained the home for herself and her daughters.

Eleanor Munsell was born in Rockly Hill, Connecticut on July 5, 1911. After graduating from Western Connecticut State College, she taught first and second grades. She married Elmer Munsell in late 1935 and spent her married years volunteering for Red Cross and the Girl Scouts. Eleanor was active in church as an organist.

Elmer Munsell was born in Woodbury, Connecticut on January 12, 1911. He graduated from Rensselaer Polytechnic Institute in 1934 with a Chemical Engineering degree. He worked for the state of Connecticut in the Bridge Department and for the U.S. Government surveying land purchases for State Forest Developments. Until retirement in 1976, Elmer worked for T.C. Company, supervising the building of corporate office buildings and large industrial projects.

Janet Murray was born in the early 1900s and grew up in Washington, D.C. Doing crafts and caring for the people who stayed "on the home front" kept her life joyful during the long war years. She was an avid fan of Washington, its people, and its parades even though she was an experienced world traveller.

Janet Norton was born in Connecticut in 1913. She earned a BS in Art Education from Skidmore College and taught for several years. She married a young physician who, soon after their wedding, entered military service and spent the war years in the Pacific area. In 1946 he established himself in private practice in Manchester, New Hampshire, where he and Janet raised their family.

Ruth Reeves Lane was born in Missouri in 1898. Her reflections, however, took her back to her youth when she and her husband first began courting. Her poem is expressive of the harmony found by many in those earlier years.

Dorothy Ryan was born in 1888. In the centennial year of her birth, she was kind enough to reflect back on one of her favorite sports. When the resulting baseball cap of words was presented to her for approval, she was thrilled.

Mark Spies, born in 1904 in Illinois, is now wheelchair bound and very frail. With his lovely wife, Mary, by his side, he was, however, able to tell us about his great love for roses. Several years ago he engineered and developed the prize-winning miniature rose now called "Cupcake" by horticulturists.

Marie Detrick Sprigg, born in Ohio in 1901, is a woman full of memories. The tales she tells of her childhood take us back to the days of parlors, and backyard stoops, and homemade ice cream. Her two contributions seem full of sunshine and good times.

Ellen Thomas, born in 1892, in Mississippi, gave us a series of little thoughts about life in the 20th century: country schoolhouses, ice chests, and quilting bees. Her true loyalties, however, lie with her wonderful husband, now gone, and her children and grandchildren.

Frances Quinn Trapp was born in 1901 in Pennsylvania. She married a Washingtonian in 1932 and has lived in the metropolitan area ever since. She tells us that, although she never worked outside the home, she had a full time job raising five children, three of whom are still living. Mrs. Trapp's primary interests are people and reading. Always reading!

Helen Escha Tyler is a writer of some repute. She published five books and has written both folk tales and a biography. Her memory of the late 1800s and early 1900s is vivid and brings to mind much of value in the lives of people in that less hurried era.

Marymount University graduate students involved in the process:*

Wendy Campbell was born in California, grew up in a military family, living both in Europe and Japan and throughout the United States. In 1968, she married Lawson "Skip" Campbell, had two sons, now 14 and 17, and currently lives in McLean, VA, where she is teaching second grade for Fairfax County. Her avocations are medieval re-creation and doll collecting.

Nan Cooper was born Nancy Anna Hammond in North Carolina where she subsequently attended the University of North Carolina at Greensboro. She also married in 1968 and has two sons. She enjoys working with children, was an Arlington County School Crossing Guard for 6 years, and is now teaching fourth grade. Her hobbies include Cub Scouts and PTA.

Kathy Koczyk, being born at Ft. Devens, Massachusetts, calls herself "kind of an Army brat." She has traveled extensively, spending time in Kyoto, Japan. In her early teens, she started teaching swimming and later extended that to other subjects. She currently directs extended day care in Arlington, VA.

---

*Note: All the students have received the Master of Educaton degree since the recording of the stories.

Jan Vincent was born in Detroit, Michigan. She received a BA in history from University of Corpus Christi in Texas in January of 1970. Jan worked for Fairfax County Public Schools prior to pursuing her MEd which she received from Marymount University in June, 1988. She is currently employed as an elementary school teacher in Fairfax County.

Some stories were provided for students that were not really useable. The students' names are included because they presented lessons and helped considerably with the project, but there are no stories directly attributed to interpretation of the students.

Alice Paxton attended Okaloosa-Walton Junior College in Niceville, FL and received her BA from American University in Sociology. In May, 1989, she received her Master's in Education from Marymount University. Alice and her family recently moved to Ft. Campbell, Kentucky.

Linda Trossback was born in Massachusetts where she has spent summers and likes to vacation. She has an undergraduate degree in philosophy from Vanderbilt University and enjoys teaching upper grades. She "always sees the glass half full!"

Lynn Wilker is from Bellevue, PA, where she was born. She attended the University of Pittsburgh, graduating Magna Cum Laude and received her Master's in Education from Marymount University in 1988. Lynn has been noted for her superior writing skills in all of her endeavors. She is now residing in Virginia Beach, Virginia.

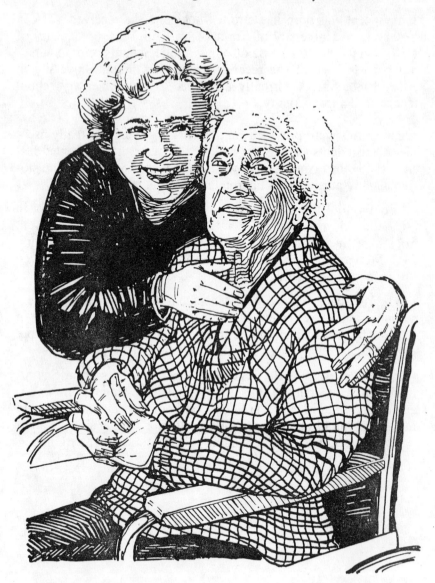

Appendix A

The materials provided in this appendix give the flavor of several instructional sessions. The materials are not complete; that is, they do not contain all the hand-outs, question sequences used, nor all the media needed to present any one full session. What the mental stimulation examples do contain are a variety of puzzles, a circle the word sample, a flow chart, an echo play, and check lists. These materials were intended to provide vocabulary building and practice. The emphasis throughout the writing preparation sessions was to promote speaking and responding to words and stories. Perhaps the examples will provide ideas for other volunteers who wish to encourage elderly people to write about the interesting events that have happened during their lifetime.

The participants at the nursing center enjoyed the echo play and produced it for a number of guests. There were costumes and many comments about the characters that performed and the characters they were representing.

The group at Countryside Manor who examined the pollution materials was intrigued by the idea of the pollution of the mind and the pollution of time. Ideas were generated by them about the way in which these types of pollution could take place.

Both groups enjoyed the stories or biographical sketches of people who had contributed to our country's past. A sample of information about Davy Crockett and a circle-the-answer worksheet about Johnny Appleseed is given here. Several more were developed in other sessions.

TEACHING AND LOVING THE ELDERLY
(A sample instructional session plan)

MENTAL STIMULATION

"Wonders of Western North America" filmstrip/tape from National Geographic Society.

Purpose: To reacquaint the participants with the beauty of the West
and the natural wonders that one can see and enjoy there.

Behavioral Objectives:

1. Given the song "Home on the Range", the participants will
   predict what we will be studying about today.
2. Given the filmstrip, the participants will attend.
3. Given the story "Wind, Sand, and Sky," the participants will
   attend.
4. Given the song, "I'm Goin' to Leave Ole Texas Now," the
   participants will take part.
5. Given the song, "Covered Wagons," the participants will
   participate.
6. Given the song, "When It's Springtime in the Rockies," the
   participants will take part.
7. Given a story about the Grand Canyon, the particpants will
   read it for "roomwork."

Procedure

Opener: The scene will open with the "Grand Canyon Suite" playing. The participants will then sing "Home on the
Range."

Learning Experiences:

The participants will:

1. View the filmstrip and listen to the tape "Wonders of Western
   North America."
2. Answer the following questions:

   How many of you have visited the West?
   What does Rio Grande mean? (big river)
   What were the "stone logs" called? (petrified)
   How many geysers are there in Yellowstone: 100; 1,000; or
   (10,000)?
   What can be found in the Sequoia National Park? (redwood
   trees)
   What is the name of the highest mountain in North Amer-
   ica? (McKinley)

3. Listen to the story, "Wind, Sand, and Sky."
4. Sing "I'm Going to Leave Ole Texas Now."
5. Learn to sing "Covered Wagons."
6. Sing "Springtime in the Rockies."
7. Be given "roomwork."

Summary and Challenge:

Emphasize the beauty of the vast land we have studied and plan for more detailed study of the spacial areas of the West.

Evaluation:

Note participation in the singing.

Materials:

"Wonders of Western North America" filmstrip/tape from National Geographic Society.

Transparencies for all the songs.

FIGURE 1. Sample block puzzle.

WESTERN NORTH AMERICA

The West coast of North America has many fine examples of natural wonders. There is splendor in the huge rock formations in Bryce and Zion Canyons. The Grand Canyon is an awe-inspiring sight. The power of wind and water are very clearly displayed in this wonder. From Yellowstone Park to Mt. McKinley to Crater Lake the unusual works of nature can be seen in the West.

1. Devil's Tower and Devil's Post piles can be found in _____.
2. Half Dome faces this valley.
3. This place is truly Grand.
4. This wood is very hard and the trees it comes from are Giants.
5. In New Mexico, We have Carlsbad _____.
6. A Lake created by a volcanic eruption.
7. Scientists who study the earth.

FIGURE 1. Answer sheet.

WESTERN NORTH AMERICA

The West coast of North America has many fine examples of natural wonders. There is splendor in the huge rock formations in Bryce and Zion Canyons. The Grand Canyon is an awe-inspiring sight. The power of wind and water are very clearly displayed in this wonder. From Yellowstone Park to Mt. McKinley to Crater Lake the unusual works of nature can be seen in the West.

1.	W	y	O	M	i	N	G	
2.	y	O	S	E	M	i	T	E
3.	C	A	N	y	O	N		
4.		R	E	D	W	O	O	D
5.		C	A	V	E	R	N	S
6.	C	R	A	T	E	R		
7.	G	E	O	L	O	G	I	S	T	S

1. Devil's Tower and Devil's Post piles can be found in _____.
2. Half Dome faces this valley.
3. This place is truly Grand.
4. This wood is very hard and the trees it comes from are Giants.
5. In New Mexico, We have Carlsbad _____.
6. A Lake created by a volcanic eruption.
7. Scientists who study the earth.

FIGURE 2. Sample vocabulary list for Western North American session.

VOCABULARY

EROSION:

STALACTITES:

GLACIER:

HABITAT:

GEOLOGICAL   FORMATIONS:

FIGURE 3. Sample traditional crossword puzzle.

R O C K Y   M O U N T A I N S

CROSSWORD PUZZLE CLUES

ACROSS

1.   A staple crop raised in Idaho.

3.   Means "of" in Spanish.

5.   An artificial watering process.

7.   This geographic feature divides the continent.

9.   A big crop in the Northwest.

11. Many small _____ make a river.

13. The mile-high city.

15. A sweet crop.

17. A canyon that is known to be great.

19. The metal used for turquoise jewelry.

21. A park with large rock formations.

23. This means green mesa.

DOWN

2.   A shiny, reddish metal.

4.   A strong storm accompanied by thunder and lightening.

6.   Add, subtract, _____ and multiply.

8.   This was discovered in California in 1848.

10. Sharp, high mountains in Wyoming.

12. The informal name for the Rocky Mountains.

14. Dodge City, Kansas, was the end of the _____ drive.

16. One of the crops raised in California. Corned beef and _____.

18. The short name for Latter Day Saints of Jesus Christ.

20. Old Faithful is a famous _____.

22. The Rockies are young _____.

24. A second rock canyon in Utah.

26. A valuable mineral needed for lasers/x-rays, etc.

FIGURE 3. (continued) Rocky Mountain crossword puzzle.

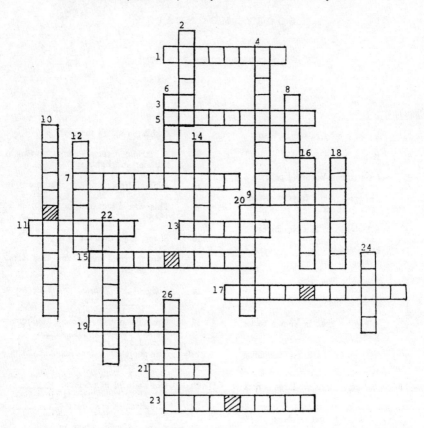

FIGURE 3. Answer sheet.

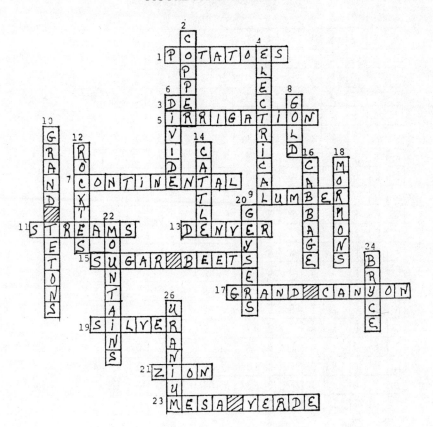

FIGURE 4. Circle the word example.

M	P	Z	G	X	Q	A	R	L	N	A	V	A	J	O
N	E	O	R	P	B	Q	R	S	B	E	A	R	S	T
U	T	S	E	V	I	W	T	R	A	I	L	S	X	Y
Z	R	P	A	A	G	B	Y	C	D	E	L	F	G	H
I	I	H	T	V	B	C	W	I	L	D	L	I	F	E
W	F	O	S	K	E	J	O	S	H	U	A	Z	A	J
A	I	T	M	R	N	R	B	R	O	C	H	U	R	E
B	E	O	O	A	D	C	D	E	S	C	E	N	I	C
H	D	G	K	P	F	G	H	E	P	I	C	J	K	L
C	F	R	Y	L	M	N	O	P	H	Q	N	R	E	S
R	O	A	M	A	T	N	O	S	I	B	E	U	N	V
A	R	P	T	N	W	N	X	Y	L	Z	D	A	O	B
E	E	H	S	O	O	C	D	B	A	E	N	F	T	G
T	S	G	U	I	D	E	S	O	D	A	E	B	S	R
A	T	C	Z	T	D	E	I	R	E	F	P	G	W	E
C	H	D	E	A	T	H	V	A	L	L	E	Y	O	I
I	I	J	K	N	L	M	N	X	P	U	D	O	L	C
L	W	I	N	D	C	A	V	E	H	T	N	D	L	A
E	C	A	L	I	F	O	R	N	I	A	I	Q	E	L
D	V	I	S	I	T	O	R	S	A	H	R	S	Y	G

BIG BEND	UTAH	ZION	CALIFORNIA
WIND CAVE	MESA VERDE	BORAX	SCENIC
BEARS	INDEPENDENCE HALL	GLACIER	GUIDES
BISON	PHILADELPHIA	DELICATE ARCH	NAVAJO
VISITORS	BRYCE	YELLOWSTONE	WILDLIFE
NATIONAL PARK	BROCHURE	TRAILS	PETRIFIED FOREST
GREAT SMOKY MTS.	DEATH VALLEY	JOSHUA	PHOTOGRAPH

TEACHING AND LOVING THE ELDERLY
(An instructional session dealing with endangered species)

*Note: There were several sessions on this general topic.

MENTAL STIMULATION

"Africa's Imperiled Paradise," Filmstrip and tape from the National Geographic Society.

Purpose: To examine the problem of endangered species on a broader scale than just U.S. species.

Behavioral Objectives:

1. Given an opportunity to put on a play, the particpants will present "Fire Bringer."
2. Given the introduction to Africa the participants will listen.
3. Given the filmstrip "Africa, Imperiled Paradise," the participants will attend.
4. Given two maps, the participants will assist in locating the Serengeti and other game parks.
5. Given a series of questions the participants will discuss the filmstrip.
6. Given a puzzle of Tanzania, the participants will fill in the missing words.
7. Given an assignment, the participants will read about Mikumi National Park for the presentation next week.
8. Given an opportunity to sing, the participants will sing "Kum Ba Yah."

Procedure:

Opener

Review the ideas from the previous week including "Fire Bringer." Prepare for the "African Safari."

Learning Experiences

1. Participants will "put on" the play, "Fire Bringer," dealing with an endangered species in America.
2. A verbal introduction and transition to African endangered species will be made.
3. Filmstrip, "Africa, Imperiled Paradise" will be shown.
4. The location of the Serengeti and other game parks will be shown on maps.
5. Questions about the filmstrip:

   a. Name 5 animals that have survived from the Stone Age. (rhino, elephant, ostrich, giraffe, hippo)
   b. Why did these animals survive?
   c. What causes the long distance migrations of animals in Africa? (search for water and good grazing)
   d. How large is the Serengeti game park? (5,000 sq. miles)
   e. Which animal needs suntan oil? (hippo)

6. Present the puzzle.
7. Hand out the Mikumi "homework."
8. Sing "Kum Ba Yah."

Summary and Futuristic Challenge

When you come next week, we'll learn more about the fantastic imperiled animals of Africa, and we'll learn about some of the customs of the people who live in several African countries.

Evaluation

1. Note the number of questions answered.
      1   2   3   4   5   6
2. Note participation in puzzle and singing.

Name: _____

Participated	Participated but	Was not willing to	Did Not
Eagerly	Needed Help	Participate, But	Follow
		Listened	

Materials:

Filmstrip:	"Africa: Imperiled Paradise"
Crossword:	Tanzania, Africa"
Reading:	*Mikumi National Park* and questions
Maps:	World Map, two maps of Africa (overheads)
Reading:	From National Geographic: "Africa"
Song:	Kum Ba Yah (on overhead)

ECHO PLAY

(Sample echo play structure that can be used with any topic)

FIRE BRINGER*
* Adapted from the book *The Fire Bringer: A Paiute Indian Legend*
as retold by Margaret Hodges, illustrated by Peter Parnall. Boston,
MA: Little, Brown and Co. 1972.

Characters:

> INDIAN BOY
> COYOTE (Counselor)
> First Man
> Second Man
> Third Man
> Spirit of the Sky
> Spirit of the Fire

Instructions for Putting on the play:
Costumes:

Indian boy:	Wears his pants legs rolled up, and and an apron out of two pieces of construction paper.
Coyote:	White sheet, and at the end, add strips of yellow paper to sheet.
1st, 2nd, and 3rd man:	If girls, they will wear white sheets with a belt around the waist. Boys

	will wear white shirts with strings tied around it, and their pant legs rolled up.
Spirit of the Sky:	Will wear regular clothes, but will be out of sight.
Spirit of the Fire:	Placed out of sight, wearing regular clothes, near the fan of fire.

Setting:

Takes place in a time long ago before fire was brought to the tribes, when men and beast could talk together, and understand each other.

Setting between scenes:

At the first stop—have a cover with black construction paper on the wall for the darkness, purple paper cut into mountain shapes.

At the second stop—white paper on the floor for the dessert and green strips of paper for the grass.

Third stop—brown paper cut into hill shaped pieces placed on the wall, and trees cut out of cardboard.

The stick will have a red and yellow paper on it.

The play itself

ECHO PLAY

THE FIRE BRINGER

Scene I—The Two are Alone

INDIAN BOY:	My people suffer and have no way to escape the cold.
ECHO:	My people suffer and have no way to escape the cold.
COYOTE:	I have fur skin and cannot feel the cold.
ECHO:	I have fur skin and cannot feel the cold.

INDIAN BOY:	Help us to keep warm.
ECHO:	Help us to keep warm.
COYOTE:	It will be hard, but we will go west and bring fire from the Burning Mountain.
ECHO:	It will be hard, but we will go west and bring fire from the Burning Mountain.
INDIAN BOY:	How will know the fire? O Spirit of the Sky, Help us.
ECHO:	How will know the fire? O Spirit of the Sky, Help us.
Spirit of the Sky:	You will need one hundred strong men and women, and three swift runners. You will know when you reach the fire.
ECHO:	You will need one hundred strong men and women, and three swift runners. You will know when you reach the fire.
INDIAN BOY:	I will find the runners.
ECHO:	I will find the runners.

Scene II — Move to another part of the room.

COYOTE:	All swift runners will walk beside me, others will follow. (They began to walk.)
ECHO:	All swift runners will walk beside me, others will follow. (They began to walk.)
Spirit of the Sky:	O Counselor, you will leave one man here in the woods, choose him now.
ECHO:	O Counselor, you will leave one man here in the woods, choose him now.
COYOTE:	You — first runner will wait here.
ECHO:	You — first runner will wait here.
1st Man:	How will I know when I see the fire?
ECHO:	How will I know when I see the fire?
COYOTE:	It is red like a flower, but it is not a flower.
ECHO:	It is red like a flower, but it is not a flower.

Spirit of the Sky:	Move on soon and leave another man at the desert.
ECHO:	Move on soon and leave another man at the desert.
COYOTE:	I will do so. (They walk on.) Second runner wait here
ECHO:	I will do so. Second runner wait here
2nd Man:	Is the fire a beast?
ECHO:	Is the fire a beast?
COYOTE:	No, and you must not let it touch the grass.
ECHO:	No, and you must not let it touch the grass.
Spirit of the Sky:	O Counselor, move on and leave a man at the hill.
ECHO:	O Counselor, move on and leave a man at the hill.
COYOTE:	I will do so. (They walk on.) Third runner stay here until the fire comes.
ECHO:	I will do so. Third runner stay here until the fire comes.
3rd Man:	Will the fire be an enemy?
ECHO:	Will the fire be an enemy?
COYOTE:	It can be an enemy. But if you feed it with small sticks, it will keep you warm. (They walk on.)
ECHO:	It can be an enemy. But if you feed it with small sticks, it will keep you warm.
Spirit of the Sky:	Your hundred days are up—now wait for the fire.
ECHO:	Your hundred days are up—now wait for the fire.
COYOTE:	Here is the fire. (He points to the fire)
ECHO:	Here is the fire.

COYOTE:	Stay here people, I will bring a brand for the Fire Spirit.
ECHO:	Stay here people, I will bring a brand for the Fire Spirit.
COYOTE:	Guard it night and day.
ECHO:	Guard it night and day.

Scene III — Move close to the fan.

COYOTE:	I have the fire, Indian Boy!
ECHO:	I have the fire, Indian Boy!
Spirit of the Fire:	I will catch you and get my fire back. (He runs after the coyote.)
ECHO:	I will catch you and get my fire back.
COYOTE:	I dropped it. (Placing the stick down)
ECHO:	I dropped it.
INDIAN BOY:	I have it, I will take it on to the next runner. (He passes the stick on, the next runner passes it to the next and then to the third runner,)
ECHO:	I have it, I will take it on to the next runner.

Scene IV —
1st man, 2nd man,

3rd man:	"You, coyote, will be called Fire Bringer as long as you live."
ALL:	"You, coyote, will be called Fire Bringer as long as you live."

MIKUMI NATIONAL PARK
A Park in Tanzania
(Question and Answer Sample)

Many different types of animals inhabit the Mukumi Park in Southeastern Tanzania. Much of the wildlife which inhabits the well-wooded water courses can be seen in the plain from time to time. However, if you take the 'River Drive' from near the Hippo

Pool towards the main road, you are likely to see wildebeest and zebra in large numbers.

The wildebeest, or gnu, (Gorgon taurinus) is the 'Nyasa blue' which differs considerably from the 'white bearded' race seen in the northern parks of Tanzania. Although the general appearance of the breeds is much alike, the 'Nyasa blue' is unbearded and much paler in body color, with the result that its stripes show up very clearly. A small percentage have a white 'chevron' across the muzzle a few inches below the eyes.

Both races, known as NYUMBU in Swaziland, are rather ungainly looking creatures much given to frolicking about, expecially when excited. A mature male weighs about 500 pounds and measures 52 inches at the shoulder. The calves, for the first few months of their lives, are a light fawn, while the adults are a brownish-grey with dark streaks and stripes across the back. Their legs are a dark tan. Wildebeest are entirely gazers but are not afraid to venture into sparsely wooded areas in search of succulent grass. They are very gregarious animals, often associating in large herds in common with zebra.

Burchell's zebra (Equus Burchelli) appears to the casual observer to move about in large homogeneous herds, but in reality is divided into family groups of up to a dozen animals, led by a dominant stallion. As the young males reach maturity, they break away from the family until such time as they are able to establish their own, either by enticing young mares away from other groups or, on occasion, by taking over a ready-made unit either by conquest or as replacement of a stallion which has become too old or has been taken by predators. A zebra stallion may stand 12 hands and weigh around 600 pounds; the females are slightly bigger.

Young zebra, looking for all the world like stuffed toys, have brownish-red stripes for the first few months of their lives.

Yellow baboons, (Papio cynocephalus, NYANI in Swahili) are commonly seen near the river banks as they feed in the trees or forage in the grassland for roots, insects, grubs and palatable vegetable material. This baboon species is lighter in both color and build than the Olive baboon, seen in northern Tanzania, and has less bushy hair on the cheeks and shoulders.

Troupes of baboons are usually controlled by a dominant male with, next in the hierarchy, three or four fully mature animals, also males, who keep on the fringes of the group as it moves across country in search of food. The young, as is the case with most primates, are rather helpless for the first few weeks of life and are carried under their mothers' chests and cling to the fur, but later often ride on their mothers' backs, perched rather far back like a man riding a donkey.

A baboon troupe is rarely silent except when fully engrossed in feeding. The sub-adults seem to obtain great pleasure from teasing those younger and smaller than themselves, and it is a common sight to see some young creature, screaming pitifully, hanging at the exteme tip of a flimsy tree limb while another tries to shake him loose. Should the dominant male be nearby, however, he is likely to cuff both offender and offended indiscriminately, causing a further outbreak of frightened screaming, as the group leaders are, or attempt to be, great disciplinarians.

MIKUMI TEST
(Sample questions for participants to complete about Mikumi National Park)

1. What is the name of the National Park you have just read about?
2. Describe the 'Nyasa blue' wildebeest?
3. What is the size of the male wildebeest?
4. Tell about the wildebeest eating habits.
5. The homogeneous looking groups of zebra are not really just huge herds. What can you tell about the herd?
6. What is the size of the zebra female?
7. What is the food of the baboon?
8. How is the baboon troupe governed?
9. How are the young baboon cared for?
10. Describe young baboon behavior.

MIKUMI ANSWER SHEET
(Sample answer sheet for instructor use)

1. Mikumi
2. Unbearded and pale color (brownish-grey); stripes can be clearly seen.
3. Weight 500 pounds, and measures over 4 feet at the shoulder.
4. Grazers, they go into the wooded areas to get succulent grasses.
5. The heard is divided into family groups, led by a dominant stallion.
6. Weight 600 pounds, 12 hands high, female larger.
7. Roots, insects, grubs and vegetables.
8. Dominant male, with 3 or 4 mature males guard the fringes of the troupe as it moves from place to place.
9. Carried about by the mother on her chest — later on her back.
10. Love to tease and play practical jokes on each other.

TEACHING AND LOVING THE ELDERLY
(Sample science instructional session plan)

PLACES WHERE PLANTS AND ANIMALS LIVE
Fimlstrip/tape: *"The Stream"* by National Geographic Society

I. *Purpose*: To acquaint the participants with the stream and with the plants and animals that can be found around it. This will serve as the beginning of the sessions on environmental pollution.

II. *Behavioral Objectives*:

1. Given a filmstrip/tape on "The Stream," the participants will attend.
2. Given a detailed map of the United States, the participants will locate rivers; and will identify the directional part of the country in which these rivers are found.
3. Given a List Poem beginning, the participants will describe a stream.
4. Given a story starter, the participants will volunteer to tell "a

fish story,'' or a ''shooting the rapids,'' or a ''skinny dip-
ping'' story.

5. Given an ideational fluency test item ''Crossing the Stream,''
   the participants will do a 2 minute rapid fire of all the ideas
   that come to mind.
6. Given information about pollution of water and streams, the
   participants will attend.
7. Given an example of air pollution, the participants will cover
   the information together while the teacher reads it orally.
8. Given several songs about rivers and streams, the participants
   will join in the singing.
9. Given ''roomwork,'' the participants will read the information
   on environmental pollution.

III. *Procedure*:

A. Opener: Verbally introduce the filmstrip. Indicate that they
   will need to note details like animal and insect names.

B. Learning Experiences: The participants will:

   1. View the filmstrip.
   2. Examine the map of the U.S.; some participants will help
      trace the major rivers in the United States.
   3. Write a List Poem under the direction of the teacher.
   4. Tell ''fish stories,'' or other stream adventures.
   5. Produce ideas about ''Crossing the Stream.''
   6. Examine information about water pollution.
   7. Review information about pollution as teacher guides them.
   8. Sing songs about rivers and streams.
   9. Receive ''roomwork'' about pollution.

C. Summary and Future Challenge

   Provide a verbal summary of the work done on ''The stream''
   and challenge the participants with the topic of ''The Woods''
   for the next time.

IV. *Evaluation*: Note the degree of participation in the tracing of
the rivers, in the List Poem and in the singing.

FIGURE 5. Simple checklist for participants to use in outdoor walks.

Atmosphere

What did you see when you looked at the sky?

Blue, clear sky □   Cloudy □   Hazy □
Rainy □   Snow □   Smoke from stacks □

Soil and Rocks

What types of soil did you see?

Dark and rich □   Sandy □   Clay □
Hardpack and bare □   Bare □
Scarcely covered □   Covered with vegetation □

List types of vegetation:

_____

_____

_____

Biosphere

What living things did you see?

1.   What types of plants and trees grow here?

      Plants:
      Grasses □   Small bushes and shrubs □
      Flowers □   Hay or grains □

      What types of flowers grow here?

      List three types.

      _____

      _____

      _____

      Trees:
      Birches □   Cedars □   Pines and firs □
      Maples □   Oaks □   Elms □

Water

What water did you see?

Type:
Ocean ☐   Lake ☐   Pond ☐
River ☐   Stream ☐   Fountain ☐

Water movement:
Rapid ☐   Sluggish ☐   Trickle ☐
Stagnant ☐

Appearance:
Clean ☐   Brown ☐   Murky ☐
Green with Algae ☐   Black and thick ☐

Refuse:
None ☐   Some around edges ☐
Floating away from shore ☐   Clogged with refuse ☐

Is any method used to keep water pure?

Screens ☐   Chlorination ☐   Aeration ☐
Pipes ☐   Forced air ☐   Bed of stones ☐
Other ☐

Man-made Items

What man-made things did you see?

Means of transportation:
Cars ☐   Streetcars ☐   Bicycles ☐
Motorbikes ☐   Buses ☐   Planes ☐
Trains ☐   Horses ☐   Subway ☐
Other ☐

Industrial sites:
Clothing ☐   Steel mills ☐   Canning ☐
Shoes ☐   Oil refineries ☐   Car ☐
Pulp mills ☐   Chemical plants ☐   Other ☐

Dwellings:
Homes ☐   Duplex ☐   Condos ☐
Farm ☐   Apartments ☐   Townhouses ☐

Stores:
Clothing ☐   Drug stores ☐   Furniture ☐
Food ☐   Hardware ☐   Restaurant ☐
Sports ☐   Music ☐   Book ☐
Video ☐   Cookie ☐   Other ☐

FIGURE 5 (continued)

2.   What type of vertebrae live here?

Birds:
Pigeons ☐   Swallows ☐   Crows ☐
Sparrows ☐   Robins ☐   Chickens ☐
Bluejays ☐   Pheasants ☐   Other ☐

Reptiles:
Snakes ☐

Amphibians:
Frogs ☐   Salamanders ☐   Toads ☐

Mammals:
Squirrels ☐   Mice, rats ☐   Deer ☐
Chipmunks ☐   Rabbits ☐   Skunks ☐
People ☐

Number of people in your range of vision:
Over 200 ☐   50-200 ☐   Under 50 ☐

Types:
Herbivores ☐   Omnivores ☐   Carnivores ☐

Fish:
Hatcheries ☐   Fish ladders ☐   Other ☐

List living fish:

_____

_____

_____

3.   What other types of living things did you see?

Insects:
Mosquitoes ☐   Spiders ☐   Ticks ☐
Flies ☐   Fleas ☐   Bees/hornets ☐

FIGURE 6. Flow chart sample for use in organizing and sharpening thinking skills.

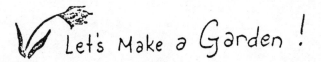

Let's Make a Garden!

Below are listed the steps in making a garden
Put this list in order and fill in the
chart.
• Buy packages of seeds.
• Prepare ground for planting.
• Plant seeds.
• Measure for planting.
• Decide what and when to plant.
• Water seeds after planting.
• Fertilize the ground.

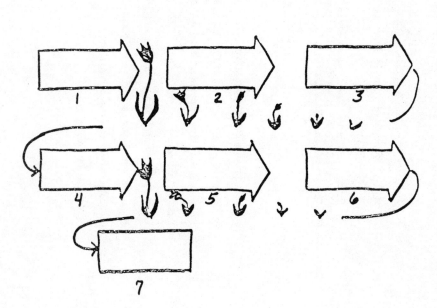

FIGURE 7. Sample of a puzzle where the true/false circled answer provides a name.

Instructions:

Circle the answer to each statement as though the letters next to the phrases were T(true) or F(false). When you finish the puzzle you should have spelled out the last name of a famous person. Write his name in the blanks beside the name Johnny.

JOHNNY _____

	T	F
John Chapman planted apple groves	A	F
Appleseed was the first name of Chapman's son	M	P
To get a special type of apple, grafting is done	P	O
Johnny Appleseed was born in Ohio	Q	L
There are many apple groves in Ohio and Indiana	E	R
John Chapman always brought a Bible with him	S	P
Chapman moved about in a big wagon	N	E
Apples are an excellent food	E	U
John Chapman is a folk hero	D	L

V. *Materials*:
- Filmstrip/tape: "The Stream," in "Places Where Plants and Animals Live" from National Georgaphic Society Educational Filmstrips.
- Transparencies of songs.
- Transparencies of List Poem beginning, "Crossing the Stream."
- Roomwork handouts

TOPIC: POLLUTION
(Sample topic examined in environmental pollution materials)

Subtopics
Air pollution
Water pollution
Earth pollution
Noise pollution
Pollution of living things
Pollution of time
Pollution of the mind

Select one subtopic
Air pollution

The following schema will give an introduction to the sources of air pollution, its sources as well as proposed solutions. Much more development is needed in each cell of the matrix, and the expansion of the data in the matrix becomes the basis for research. For example, polluted air in turn pollutes water, land and living things, and this can be researched in another, later phase of the research.

MATRIX		AIR POLLUTION
POLLUTERS	SOURCES OF POLLUTION	POSSIBLE SOLUTIONS
People	Cars Oil burners Burning waste	1. Develop awareness 2. Walk, use bikes, join car pool

		3. Do not burn waste
		4. Use electric heat
Community and city	Industry Mass transportation	1. Create air pollution laws 2. Create mass transit system (e.g., electric cars)
	Burning Waste	3. Create better method to dispose of waste
National and International Companies	Industry	1. Designate funds for research to develop pollution controls
	Destruction of national forests	2. Create more national parks, reforest large areas
	Use of poisonous gases	3. Change priorities from war to universal survival
	International transport	4. Get international anti-pollution laws

MATRIX		WATER POLLUTION
POLLUTERS	SOURCES OF POLLUTION	POSSIBLE SOLUTIONS
People	Waste products Fishing equipment	1. Develop awareness 2. Place waste in containers 3. Use safe equipment
Community and city	Sewage Improper Land Fills	1. Properly process sewage 2. Use approved land fill process
National and	Waste Materials	1. Provide funds for proper waste disposal

International Companies	Toxic Wastes Oil Spills	2. Create toxic waste dumps
		3. Get laws requiring safe transport of oil products
		4. Have laws enforced

SAM HOUSTON
(Sample of information about a great American and accompanying puzzle)

General Sam Houston was a tall man. The exact height does not seem clear, but people always said he was taller than anyone else around. He was about 6 feet 6 inches, far taller than the average man in those days.

Sam was born on March 2, 1793 in Virginia. He had four older brothers, one younger brother and three sisters. His father was a military man. Sam learned to read at home and did not like school, so he didn't attend. He liked to pretend to do big things like perhaps be a Revolutionary soldier; he loved stories of heroes.

The family moved to Tennessee when Sam was thirteen. Sam's father sold the Virginia farm and bought 419 acres of land in Tennessee, but before the move was begun, Sam's father died. Mrs. Houston told the boys to pack up the wagons; they would go anyway.

Sam did not like clearing territory and plowing land all day long. By the time he was fourteen, he headed West. He lived with Cherokee Indians for three years.

He fought and was seriously wounded in the War of 1812. After the Battle of Horseshoe Bend, Sam was left all night on the battlefield because the doctors said that he wouldn't last the night. He had a huge arrow wound in the groin, two shots in the shoulder and one in the arm. He did last the night, however, and finally recovered fully although it took him over a year to do so.

Sam Houston stayed in the army and was promoted to become an officer. He had a disastrous marriage, and left the settled lands to move into unsettled territory when he was about 35 years old. He returned to the Cherokee people he loved and married a princess, Tiana.

Finally at 39 he moved into Texas where he was soon drawn into politics and the maelstrom of the war for independence for Texas. He was wounded again and had continuing problems with old wounds. He did recover enough to be elected the first President of the Texas Republic. He died on July 26, 1863 having served his country in many ways.

FIGURE 8. Sample Computer generated puzzle.

TEXAS

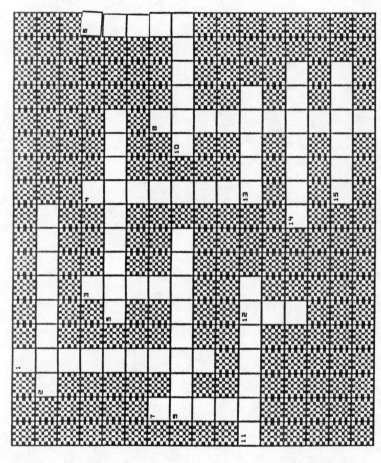

FIGURE 8 (continued)

ACROSS CLUES

2. A BEAR KILLER
5. THE RIVER THAT SEPARATES TEXAS
   AND MEXICO
9. THE NICKNAME OF TEXAS
10. A CITY WHERE A PRESIDENT WAS
    KILLED
11. THE NAME OF THE FIRST PRESIDENT
    OF TEXAS
13. HOUSTON'S INDIAN WIFE
14. THE OCCUPATION OF MANY TEXAS MEN
15. THE COUNTRY THAT WANTED TO KEEP
    TEXAS

DOWN CLUES

1. SAM HOUSTON WAS THE FIRST
3. HOUSTON HAD ----- CHILDREN
4. THE MOTHER OF HOUSTON'S CHILDREN
6. THE NAME OF THE STATE
7. REMEMBER THE
8. THE ALAMO WAS NEAR THE CITY OF
12. A PRODUCT THAT TEXAS IS WELL
    KNOWN FOR

WORD LIST: TEXAS

ALAMO
COWBOYS
CROCKETT
DALLAS
EIGHT

HOUSTON
LONESTAR
MARGARET
MEXICO
OIL

PRESIDENT
RIOGRANDE
SANANTONIO
TIANA
XAS

ANSWERS: TEXAS

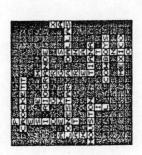

Suggested Readings

Andrews, Theodore E., Houston, W. Robert, and Bryant, Brenda L. (1981). *ADULT LEARNERS (A RESEARCH STUDY)*. Washington, DC: Association of Teacher Education.

John, Martha Tyler. (1988). *GERAGOGY: A THEORY FOR TEACHING THE ELDERLY*. New York, NY: The Haworth Press, Inc.

John, Martha Tyler. (1983). *TEACHING AND LOVING THE ELDERLY*. Springfield, IL: Charles C. Thomas.

Knowles, Malcolm. (1975). *SELF-DIRECTED LEARNING*. New York, NY: Association Press.

Koch, Kenneth. (1977). *I NEVER TOLD ANYBODY*. New York, NY: Vintage Books.

Nessel, Denise D., Jones, Margaret B., Dixon, Carol N. (1989). *THINKING THROUGH THE LANGUAGE ARTS*. New York, NY: Macmillan Publishing Co.

Saul, Shura. (1983). *GROUP WORK WITH THE FRAIL ELDERLY*. New York, NY: The Haworth Press, Inc.

Smith, Christel M., and Stenger, Leslie A. *HEALTHY MOVES FOR OLDER ADULTS*. Washington, DC: ERIC Clearinghouse on Teacher Education.

Index